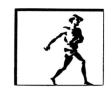

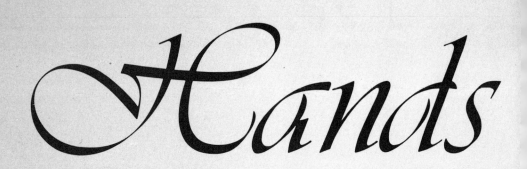

Hands

PHOTOGRAPHS BY ROBERT SWENSON
ILLUSTRATIONS BY HELEN HALL

SIMON AND SCHUSTER · NEW YORK

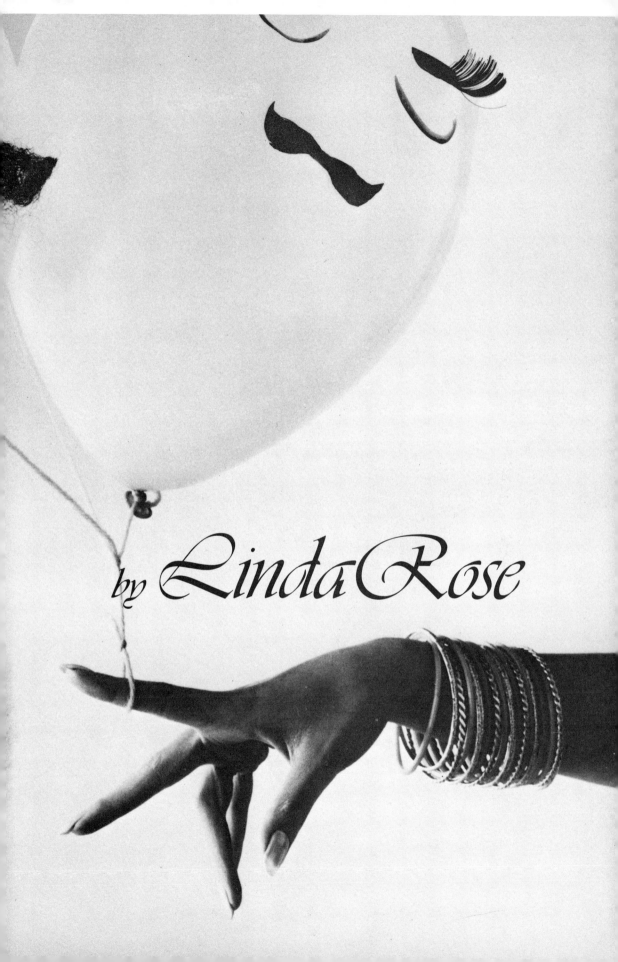

by Linda Rose

1 2 3 4 5 6 7 8 9 10

Library of Congress Cataloging in Publication Data

Rose, Linda.

Hands.

   Bibliography: p.
   1. Models, Fashion.   2. Hand—Care and hygiene.   3. Manicuring.   I. Title.
HD8039.M772U57   646.7′26   80-12204
ISBN 0-671-24944-4

Title page photograph: Stanley Johnson

Acknowledgments

2110169

I wish to acknowledge the following people who have helped me write this book:

Tanao Sands (Kumalae) for contributing valuable information from her research and writings, and for also holding up the light as well as the mirror.

Selma Evans Rose, whose motherly pride in all my efforts helped me through.

My friends Christina Crawford, Marion Gallo, John Dominic and George Cappanelli for being there.

And especially C. David Koontz, who wouldn't allow me to stray far from my path.

My agent, Susan Schulman, for her very wise choices.

Joni Evans, for inspiration and encouragement when this was only a germ of an idea.

The many people who gave me access to what seemed to be the unreachable.

And to my father, the late James Henry Rose, who had the most wonderful hands I've ever seen.

In addition, I would like to acknowledge the following professionals who have given generously of their time and expertise:

Dr. Paul Koehler of Chesebrough-Pond's, Inc.

Dr. Bry Benjamin

Dr. Norman Orentreich

Mrs. Florens Meschter

Father Edward McDonough

Hae Young, my manicurist

Tiffany and Co.

For My Sons, Peter and Danny

Contents

Hand Health and Beauty

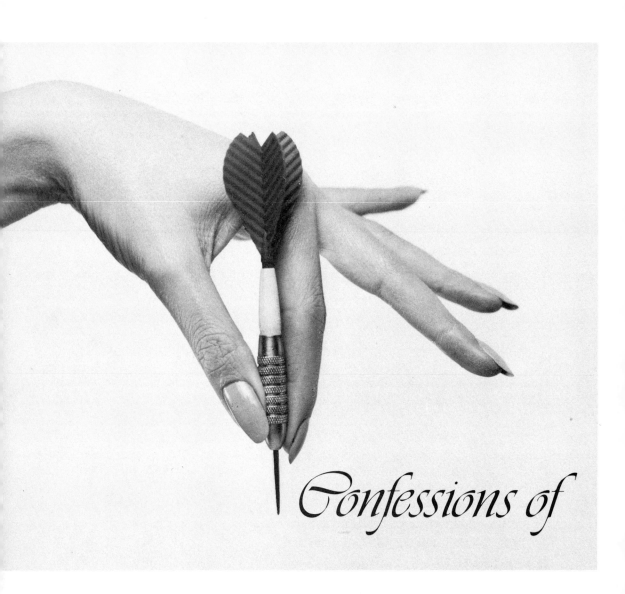

Confessions of

a Hand Model

The Business of Hands

WHAT IS IT LIKE to be a hand model in a profession where recognition of faces is a measure of success? It is not always the ego booster of all time. I used to walk onto a TV set, announce that I was the hand model and hear, "Gee, Linda, you're not such a dog!" Repeatedly in a social situation, some master of the artful put-down has introduced me to the group saying, "Meet Linda Rose. She's a model, but she just does hands." For years I was not quite sure if this technique was the ploy of the considerate hostess eager to reassure any guests who might not find the rest of me "model-worthy." Such introductions were frustrating, especially when I had fourteen commercials featuring all of me on the air.

Hand modeling is unique. It is a craft in which minute details are magnified. I have had to view hands differently from the average person; to take on the identities of famous people so that I could handle a product as if I were they. I have had to be as elegant as Lauren Hutton touching a Revlon compact or as casual as Jane Withers cleaning a sink with Comet. Hand modeling is tense, difficult and time-consuming. It is also fun, creative and very rewarding.

A hand model must have the patience of Job and nerves of steel (to say nothing of withstanding countless "hand job" jokes from people who are absolutely certain they are the first homo sapiens on the North American continent to have thought of such a clever, if suggestive, double entendre). Although usually required to report to a set at 8:30 A.M., a hand model often is the last to actually "work." Primarily this is because the makeup man, the hairdresser and the sound engineer are not necessary for your shot. Also, a testy director who is having his own problems with a nervous client often takes his troubles out on the talent. If a model has a speaking role in a commercial or is seen simply smiling on camera, she can often "act" above the tension. But unfortunately, hands are the first place nervousness shows. There isn't much of a market for shaky hands. Luckily I have never had this problem; however, I was really put to the test during a taping for a Hanes stocking ad. At the shooting the director of advertising stared into a TV monitor showing my hands holding a stocking, and instructed me how to position each of my fingers ("A little higher with the pinky, a little lower with the ring finger. Could you bend the index finger a little? Good, now hold that. I don't know."). I dutifully followed this intimidating woman's every word without a break for almost two hours. I endured this grueling torture while she argued with the director, shrieking, "I don't think those look like happy hands! Do those look like happy hands to you?" I would have gladly taken my "not so happy hands" and wrung her little neck.

If a commercial or ad isn't for nail polish or hand lotion, why would they bother with a separate model to do hands? The world of advertising realizes the importance of hands and spends an amazing amount of money each year to employ the right hands to be photographed caressing their products. For the last twenty-five years, I have done over twenty-five hundred television commercials and countless magazine ads in which only my hands were seen. Most of these ads were product shots for other women who were commercial spokeswomen—sometimes stars like Patricia Neal for Maxim or Cybill Shepherd for Clairol.

The reason for my employment was clearly that the hands touching the product were to look as good and as important as the face or personality doing the "sell." My very first commercial was for Lux soap. The director was frantically searching for someone who could simulate Gene Tierney's handwriting (across her picture as if she were signing an autograph) and also have hands befitting a star. I was doing junior fashion modeling during my summer vacations from Vassar College, and had done a stocking shot for the film company. They reasoned that if I had good legs, I might also have good hands. They also figured that if I was enrolled in college, I must have enough intelligence to forge a signature. It seems that I satisfied both requirements.

It should be noted that all the ladies whose hands I've been do not necessarily have ugly or aging hands. Often the lighting required to show off a textured lipstick case, for example, is so intense that it would magnify minute skin flaws, invisible in a natural setting. Also, there is much more skill required in product demonstration than one might imagine. Placing a tiny open compact into a miniature Christmas set without knocking anything over, with just the right timing to fit the announcer's words, imparting an elegant attitude all the while, looks simple. And it should, if done right. But in fact this work requires a steadiness and accuracy difficult for most people, even experienced performers and models.

The economics of the business dictate that it is a cash savings to have a hand expert (even though she may cost the client an extra fee often higher than that of the regular model) come in and complete one single shot rather than spend an extra hour with the star trying to get the scene done properly. As in all businesses, time is money.

In a few cases the gorgeous face the client chose has badly chewed digits. And there are always a few stars who refuse to do their own "insert work." While most stars are thrilled that a hand model is there to do some of the more sticky tasks for them (Barbara Britton used to always thank me when people complimented her TV hands) alas, a few are resentful that the client didn't find every part of them absolutely perfect. But mostly it boils down to not wanting to spend costly time where it isn't necessary, and no matter who the spokesman for the product is, the real star of the commercial is the product itself. Naturally the sponsor wants it to look its best and give it the perfect touch.

Of course there are also male hand models. Greg Fortune, who is also a spokesman and a host for game shows, is employed almost daily as the most versatile man's hand. Jan Leighton, a professional actor and master of disguises known for his wonderful portrayal as George Washington, does much hand work. Ted Madison, a black actor, handles products for Bill Cosby and Reggie Jackson. Terry Bailey, once the model for Jon Whitcomb's romantic illustrations, is probably now the most experienced hand in the business. Terry and I have passed many hours (years perhaps) working together, or at least waiting together for the spokesman or star to complete his segment of the film. During my most memorable job with Terry we spent literally three days under a table pouring Martini and Rossi wine into each other's glass. The problem was that we were placed so that we couldn't see the surface above us, and therefore were pouring "blind." I don't know if they ever got the shot they wanted, but Terry and I became very well acquainted.

Is there competition? Yes, although not so much as in regular modeling. But people are always calling me up to tell me about a niece who has really nicely shaped nails, and should she give up her apartment in Rochester for her certain career in commercials. I guess it looks much easier than it is. My favorite story about professional competition concerns the "Walking Fingers" campaign for AT&T. The creators of this very successful promotion had decided to go one "step" farther and do a "marching fingers" commercial. They held auditions for people who could not only move their fingers to the theme from *The Bridge on the River Kwai,* but also coordinate their two hands as if they were the feet of two separate marchers. The producers also needed two sets of hands that were similar so that the marching fingers all looked alike. After three days of auditioning every female hand model in New York, they matched me up with a lady who had pretty, slender fingers which seemed to be able to accomplish this crazy task. Everything was fine at the rehearsal (yes, we had to rehearse, as this was precision work), but when we went to film the actual commercial, she became tense, developed a "limp" in one finger and couldn't follow the cadence. When she also used the wrong "foot" for one take, the director despaired: "These fingers are just not good soldiers!" The spot was scrapped.

The major selling point in many commercials is, in fact, my area of expertise, i.e., the "demo," or a visible demonstration that one product is better than its competitor. Today the Federal Trade Commission carefully regulates the production of demos so that "what you see is what you get." You might not care how long it takes a pearl dropped in your shampoo to reach to the bottom of the bottle (the longer the trip, the richer the shampoo, supposedly), but at least you don't have to duplicate the experiment in your own home for verification. However, it was not always so. When I first started to work in commercials they could fudge all they wanted and usually did. When silicones were first being touted as the miraculous new protective ingredient in hand lotions, I did a commercial in which "Mennen Skin Magic" was written on the palm of my right hand, and "Brand X" on my left. Water was then rinsed over my two hands, and Brand X washed away, but Mennen Skin Magic with silicones protected my skin, as represented by the ink. The only catch was that they wrote "Mennen" with indelible ink!

My personal history book logs not only the wars of the hand lotions (Jergens' "research" methods were quite unique), the wars of the household cleaners (never one shot without added ammonia or Clorox) and laundry soap, and the ever-popular wars of the dishwashing liquids. When the FTC cracked down on the claims in these television demos, all of these product demonstrations had to be reshot under new strictly legal conditions. Lux Liquid had been using a demo in which two dirty plates were each lowered into separate Lucite tanks full of detergent, one containing Lux, and the other Brand X. Of course, as was always true in TV Land, the Lux side was clean almost instantly, while the plate dipped in Brand X was still disgustingly dirty. On the day this was to be reshot to meet the new FTC requirements, I reported to the studio and found the following: two special-effects men from Lever Brothers, countless tense agency men, clients and lawyers, and two specially built large Lucite tanks, which for some reason had no drain. It promised to be one long day, at best.

I stepped up to the Lucite tanks, received the two dishes, and on cue, with the camera rolling, dropped them neatly into the two tanks. I couldn't see what was happening because the dishes were facing the camera and this very nervous aggregation of interested parties. Suddenly a little voice from the back shouted, "Holy Mother of God, it works!" So much for truth in advertising.

Being a hand specialist allowed me to work right up to the end of my pregnancies. At the time I was doing two live shows a week for Revlon, who loyally insisted I continue to work as long as possible. The rule of thumb seemed to be that if you could still reach the table, you would do the shot. Apparently, it was so hard for agency producers to get Charlie Revson's approval on anything, much less the hands that touched his famous products, that they preferred to still use me, with all the uncertainties of advancing pregnancy, than to try to please this perfectionist with someone new. This situation became almost ludicrous when, after being hospitalized two weeks before my due date, they called to see if I could be released "just for one night." Revlon was sponsoring a new TV show called "Big Party," which was about to have its premiere. I'm sure they viewed my pregnancy and the early hospitalization as an inconvenience. Fortunately my doctor didn't spring me, because I went into labor that night. Revlon's "Big Party" and my son Peter had simultaneous debuts. It probably wouldn't have concerned Revlon if I was the first woman in history to have given birth during a live commercial as long as the pains came conveniently between shots.

Well, I've sat on a low stool, stroked a man's face with my fingers while a great beauty nuzzled her Blush On cheeks next to his (talk about feeling like a fifth wheel!), auditioned fourteen men in one hour by caressing their faces, have been wheeled around a supermarket with my hands sticking out of a grocery bag for Thrill detergent's "Buy a pair of hands" campaign, and smoothed lotion on another girl's shoulder for a new and different sociosexual experience.

I've also met hundreds of fascinating people, made excellent money and become respected nationally, if not internationally, for my craft. In the past ten years, I've been lucky enough to have been featured—all of me, that is—in over one hundred and fifty commercials, been the voice ("voice-over" in the trade) in about two hundred commercials, and hosted and co-hosted game shows and talk shows. But I still work a few days a week as a hand model. It is my special craft. What else will I ever be best at?

Shooting a TV Commercial

$\mathcal{T}$HE SHOOTING of a TV commercial usually involves the appearance of the following cast of characters:

THE PRINCIPALS, OR ACTORS, who will be seen on camera in the commercial.

THE EXTRAS: Actors who may appear in the commercial but will not be readily identifiable with the product, either because they are not in sharp focus or are seen only from the back (e.g., in some bank commercials).

THE PRODUCT DEMONSTRATOR OR HAND MODEL: The person who gets to touch or handle the product and/or perform the demonstration that shows that this product is better than its competitors.

THE MAKEUP MAN (or woman), who is hired to see that all the talent is properly made up. Often this includes hiding circles under the eyes acquired from the insomnia suffered the preceding night as a result of the anxiety attack directly related to the next day's shooting. *Note:* I rarely use hand makeup unless the cameraman wants my skin tone lighter or darker to match that of the principal actor or the requirements of the background.

THE HAIRDRESSER: The person whose job it is to keep straight hair curly (or curly hair straight) during the day's filming under unbelievably hot lights.

THE FASHION STYLIST: She (or he) is responsible for clothing the actors. She has either spent the last three days in Bloomingdale's gathering various shirtwaists, bathrobes and sweaters (the mainstay of most commercials) or the last three nights on the phone with the actors getting them to pledge in blood that they not only own, but agree to bring in, what is required for the commercial.

THE FOOD STYLIST: Often originally a graduate home economist who has refined her talents to the degree that she can not only make undercooked piecrust (for the purposes of easier cutting) look luscious (with the aid of Kitchen Bouquet), but can also duplicate a perfectly cooked rib roast or artistically browned chicken breasts for the endless number of takes required of the director (to say nothing of the acting mistakes of the talent).

THE DIRECTOR, who tells the actors where to stand, what to do, how to do it. He or she is responsible for making the commercial "come to life." Some directors specialize in "slice of life" (or "real people") commercials, while others are masters of the "tabletop" commercial, which deals mainly with the closeups of the product, such as foods. The director tells the actor where to stand (where his "marks" are), what to do, how to do it, and (best of all) he gets to yell "Action!"

THE ASSISTANT DIRECTOR (or A.D., as he is called), who sees to it that the cast and crew are ready and available to the director when he needs them. I've always suspected that the A.D., upon receiving his union card, also receives a mimeographed sheet of ten phrases to be memorized and screamed out at various times throughout the shooting day, and guaranteed to jar the ambience of the room (or set) at any time. Among these are: "Quiet on the set!"; "Makeup!"; "Hair!"; "You're late!" (screamed to an actor upon his arrival three minutes after the appointed call time); "Bells!" (which signals that a sound recording is about to be made, and sneezing during the "take" will be countered with extermination of the guilty); "Cut!" (which means "Stop the camera. The actor has eaten all of the product, or the beer is spilling all over the table); "Slate!" and/or "Sticks!" (the clapping of two wooden sticks together to synchronize the sound with the film). The commercial A.D. often gets to read the slate for the sound takes, e.g., "Take one, scene one." Very Hollywood, "One hour lunch!" (or he has to pay a union penalty to cast and crew). And finally, "It's a wrap!" meaning that the shooting day is over. This is not infrequently uttered thirty seconds before the cast and crew would be eligible for overtime pay.

THE CAMERAMAN: The director of photography, who determines how the shot is lit, and how the camera will move to get the desired effect. He also makes sure that each shot is "framed" correctly, i.e., that it includes in the picture exactly what is intended (and no more, excluding "in frame" a boom mike which often has to hover above the actors' heads, or the hand model's head or hair, when only his (or her) hands should be shown.

THE ASSISTANT CAMERAMAN, who assists the cameraman in the actual shooting. He determines the proper film exposure and actually executes the needed focus changes.

GAFFERS: The electricians who move the lights and electrical equipment.

GRIPS, who move the cameras and sets.

SET DESIGNER, who is present to see that his plans are properly carried through. Often a series of commercials for the same product will require three entirely different kitchen sets as each spot will have a different "family" cast, and therefore, advertisers reason, can't live in the same "home."

SOUND MEN: One or two men who record the commercial if dialogue is to be recorded along with the filming of the commercial.

PROPERTY MAN: The man who sees to it that all the "props" and products are ready. A hand model's best friend or worst enemy (see page 38).

THE SCRIPT SUPERVISOR, who carefully times each "take" and makes sure that each successive shot can be properly edited into the final commercial.

THE CLIENT: The owner of a company or director of advertising of the large corporation that manufactures the product being sold. He is the guy who is paying for this extravaganza. When he wants to produce a commercial he goes to an advertising agency.

THE AGENCY WRITER, who has come up with the concept as well as the actual dialogue for the commercial and will see to it that each filmed action is appropriate to his concept and words.

THE AGENCY ART DIRECTOR, who designs the visual concepts for the commercial and determines the "look" of the commercial, as it is translated to the storyboard (a series of drawings of little TV screens that depict the action as well as the titles (or "supers") that will be incorporated into the finished commercial.

THE ADVERTISING AGENCY ACCOUNT EXECUTIVE: The person who attempts to maintain a happy marriage between the agency and the client.

THE AGENCY PRODUCER: The person who casts the commercial, finds the appropriate film house, director, editor, etc., and in general the one whose ass is on the line if the various elements don't bring new meaning to the word "sales," or at least "art in advertising."

•

FAMOUS "HANDS" I'VE BEEN

Susan Blakely—Fabergé
Barbara Britton—Revlon
Kitty Carlisle—Simplicity Patterns
Gloria DeHaven—Alberto Culver Shampoo
Barbara Feldon—Revlon
Arlene Francis—Arpège
Farrah Fawcett—Fabergé
Sunny Griffin—Avon
Florence Henderson—Wesson Oil
Lauren Hutton—Revlon
Julia Meade—Kodak
Jan Miner (Madge)—Palmolive Liquid
Nico (Andy Warhol star)—Revlon
Patricia Neal—Maxim
Jennifer O'Neill—Revlon
Cybill Shepherd—Clairol
Gene Tierney—Lux soap
Jane Withers—Comet Cleanser
Gretchen Wyler—Lipton's Soup

●

HAND TALK

Hand to mouth
I have to hand it to you
Give him a hand
Out of hand
Palm it off
To finger
Handcuffed (married)
Hard as nails
Having a finger in the pie
Slap in the face
Thumb your nose at
Knuckle under
Butler's thumb
Two-fisted

Soft touch, light touch
Groping in the dark
To lift a little finger
Boardinghouse reach
Putting into safe hands
Cold hands, warm heart
Many hands make light work
Busy hands are happy hands
An iron hand in a velvet glove
A bird in the hand is worth two in the bush
One hand washes the other
The right hand doesn't know what the left hand is doing
To take your hand in marriage
To wash your hands of
At first hand
At the hands of
A backhanded compliment
In hand
On hand
Out of hand
Hand down
Hands down
Hand over
Handful
Handmade

Special Skills

AS ANYONE asked you lately if you were capable of dropping a pearl into a bottle of Prell shampoo with enough accuracy to insure that its slow trip to the bottom would be absolutely centered? Or, how long has it been since someone questioned your ability to properly burp a Tupperware container? Some shots I have been hired to do are literally as easy to accomplish as a snap (for Revlon) or making a "perfect" sign with the thumb and forefinger (for Hayleys M.O.). Usually, however, hand demos involve additional skill. In fact, more jobs are available to the hand model who has special skills like sewing (I do and have for Singer), playing piano (somewhat) and typing (not well enough for most closeups). A good legible handwriting is sometimes required for commercials, and I have written for Scheaffer Pen, Esterbrook Pen, J.C. Penney, and even Clairol. In order to be cast in these commercials, I had to not only write legibly, but also with speed and accuracy. Often my words were to take a certain number of seconds to complete as well as cover a specified amount of space for adequate camera coverage. My finest hour was when I had to write the word "slow" in ketchup for Heinz's "Slow Ketchup" campaign. I not only had to form perfect letters but also control the flow of ketchup so that the width of the "writing" was uniform. In addition, the ketchup oozed too slowly from most of the narrow-necked bottles to complete the word "slow" within the time allotted to the scene. To prepare, the Heinz people sent me home with an entire case of ketchup and paper towels so that I could learn to write "slow" fast.

THE PERFECT POUR

I'm sure that when you pour your morning coffee or your nightly beer, you cannot imagine what we go through when we pour these same products for a commercial on TV. Each liquid—soda, beer, tea, tomato juice and even cough syrups (the most viscous) —requires a different method of "pour" in order to get a precise and clean shot. By controlling the speed and angle of the bottle or can, beers are seen with just the right-sized head. Cleanliness of the glass also effects the size of head. And you must remain steady, as well as on a mark, with the pouring vessel, as it is also usually in camera view. Sometimes you have to match the speed and amount of pour with that of another hand model, who is pouring into another glass simultaneously. And, finally, it is crucial that the pour finish be "clean," that is, that absolutely no drips fall as you take the bottle out of frame. Little lapses that are easily forgiven in a home setting can be reason for divorce between client and hand model.

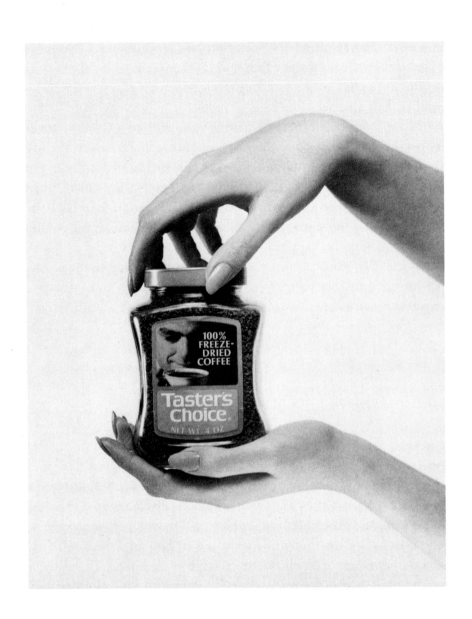

COOKING

When you slice a tomato for a commercial, the slices must not only be uniform in size all the way through the shot, but they have to fall in exactly the right position. I have carved several hundred chicken breasts for Shake and Bake in order to get just the right angle to make the juices flow freely from our hero, and not as freely from Brand X. Breaking off a piece of piecrust to properly display its flakiness before a camera can take hours of preparation and shooting. (The crust often is invisibly scored to facilitate a clean break.) I once saw a food economist who heads a testing facility for a major food company leave a film studio in tears because she just couldn't keep up with the special demands of shooting food for film. The spreading of margarine, cheese, frosting and even peanut butter all have special little styles of their own. Even a seemingly simple task like separating an egg becomes challenging when you are doing it for camera. I have learned to separate eggs with one hand as fast as a short-order cook.

Some "table-top" directors can drive you mad with insisting on take after take of the same action while they change their camera moves, frame or lighting to make sure that the shot is covered with as much variety as possible for the client. But when feature director Harold Becker was still working in commercials, the challenge to a hand model was exactly the opposite. He would set his lighting and camera moves swiftly, and then and there choose which way the shot was to be done. There was no waiting around for the clients to pick their favorite approach for him. I could never figure out whether this was the result of superconfidence in his work or a growing boredom with the job. In any case, his work was always beautiful. And he worked a lot.

His pace overwhelmed most hand models, and very few had the stamina or concentration to keep up with him. On one single day we shot the various stages of preparation of twenty-six gourmet dinners for Wesson Oil. Top food stylist Alice Kronk and I toiled in every sense of the word from 8:30 A.M. until we left at 7:30 P.M. My clothes smelled of Wesson Oil. My hair smelled of Wesson Oil. And I figured that between the two of us, we had done enough cooking to cover several years of entertaining for the busiest hostess.

FOIL

Aluminum foil and plastic wrap involve special handling. Plastic wrap can stick to itself with the slightest false move, spoiling the look of the finished product. Or it can give out—many are the heartbreaking moments when a bowl of berries that looks so neatly and securely covered is turned over and confidently shaken to demonstrate the strength when wrapped. The sight of food falling onto the studio floor while the camera rolls has been known to make grown men cry. Plastic wrap and aluminum foil must also be torn on just the correct angle or the product picture is a mess.

The visual drama of foil is that it can be molded over any shape. In one commercial, I was dramatically wrapping a new Scott aluminum foil around such diverse shapes as bread, cheese, zucchini. I was standing on my marks ready to shoot the last shot of the commercial as the food stylist handed me the truest test of all for foil, a large, perfectly wrapped-for-camera turkey. As she placed this "baby" into my carefully positioned arms, I felt the most eerie sensation. It seems that the turkey was only wrapped where the camera eye could see, and so the bottom was bare. The turkey was also raw, and the unexpected feeling of cold raw skin felt like I was cradling a three-day-old corpse.

PILL PUSHING

Commercials involving pill shots can be difficult because the objects you are handling are small, lightweight, and hard to handle with observable deliberation. Shaking out exactly two tablets from a bottle into your palm (a false bottom can be constructed making only two available on each shake) so that they fall right side up with the sponsor's trademark facing the camera is no snap.

Years ago, Bayer aspirin advertisers designed a commercial in which pills, capsules and tablets of various shapes and sizes were stacked. Different sets of hands placed one pill on top of the other, until, ideally, the last was placed on top of the stack and the camera pulled back from its extreme closeup of each hand to reveal a whole mountain of pain relievers. Although the prop man applied a tiny amount of rubber cement to the bottom of each pill so that it would stick, the stacking was at best a precarious procedure which required total dexterity and concentration on the part of the four of us hands (two male and two female models). We also had to cross to alternate sides of the tabletop set for each of our actions, being careful not to shake the table in any way. The first pills in the stack were the easiest to place. As the pile got higher, the risk of not getting your pill to stick or, worst of all, knocking down the existing stack, multiplied geometrically. Though the team spirit was terrific and we all were making an extreme effort, we couldn't get one usable take.

The two male hand models and I were working well, considering the pressures of the task, but the other lady, whom I had never seen before, was another story. She was obviously trying, but each time she touched the stack, it would crumble the perfect pile the rest of us had just made. The director gave her different-shaped pills to place, as well as different positions in the order of the pile. Nothing worked. It finally reached 5:30 P.M. and we had to call it a "wrap."

I later found out that this lady with the touch of death was actually the girl friend of one of the film company's producers. Not realizing that there might be any skill required of a hand model, he reasoned that a day's pay as a hand model might be a nice gift. It would have been cheaper to give her a diamond ring from Tiffany's, as the whole film had to be reshot another day.

Animals, Kids and Others

$\mathcal{H}$AVING TWO BABIES of my own gave me an advantage over other hand models who had no previous experience with children. At one time I did so much work with kids that it was sometimes hard to remember if I had, in fact, left home. By doing hand commercials, I have probably fed more products to children than any food-pushing Jewish grandmother. But the feeding is the easy part. It's the eating that can cause problems. Often children cast in a food commercial swear (or their mothers swear) that they love and adore the food to be featured in the spot. But when the shooting starts, the moment of truth arrives and it's often difficult to get the same supposedly eager kid to eat the likes of fried fish. That's when the stage mothers of commercial child stars go into cardiac arrest. The ensuing manipulation through bribes and threats boggles the mind.

Also, some directors just can't deal with children. I have endured hours of takes during which a director cajoles, or more frequently, bullies the child into the proper action. Years ago, on a Twinkies commercial, the child actor arrived on the set craving his share of Twinkies. Unfortunately the director insisted on so many takes that about a minute after the shot was completed, the kid threw up.

Occasionally the lack of communication between director and child can result in a seemingly endless shoot. Once, on a Fritos commercial, the child cast was no more than four years old. Although the director shot lots of film, he never got a suitable take. Finally, in total exasperation, the director walked over to the little boy, showed him the story board (approved pictures and dialogue given to the film producers by the advertising agency). He patiently explained, "Look, son, you are moving your body too close here so that I have no room for my 'super'" (title which is superimposed over the picture). The four-year-old looked at the director as if he were speaking a foreign language.

In defense of directors and producers, I must acknowledge that casting of babies and children can be terribly frustrating. Once they are lucky enough to find a child who pleases everybody involved, if a postponement of filming or a reshoot of additional scenes are needed, the lapse of time often results in a baby who just doesn't look the same as when he was cast. This can even be true when casting older children. I did an award-winning commercial for Lux liquid with an adorable five-year-old. Cindy was just darling. She appeared on camera, and I was hands and voice-over (my first). For marketing reasons, the sponsors delayed the actual airing of the commercial for a year, at which time the overwhelming positive reaction to the spot prompted the advertisers to produce a series of commercials featuring the same "family." Unfortunately, one year had changed adorable little Cindy into a six-year-old with all the sophistication of a budding Lauren Bacall. The loss of innocence resulted in the loss of a commercial for both of us.

TRYING TO HOLD THE REINS

During the course of my long career as a "manual laborer" of sorts in thousands of commercials, I have worked with dogs, horses and cats, and have even had the allegedly good-luck droppings of a white dove fall on my head while shooting a commercial for Dove soap. Pet foods are one of the largest advertisers on TV, and these spots provide lots of work for product demonstrators. In order to work successfully with animals on commercials you must be neither allergic nor scared. And the animal can't be nervous either. Most of the animals used in commercials are from a very few special animal-talent agencies. The people who run these agencies are usually reliable judges as to which animal will "work" (eat, walk on cue or sit quietly), and are experts at manipulating the animal's actions for camera.

Dog-food boxes or bags are often large and heavy, and accuracy of the pour, if not easy, is certainly crucial. If one drop of food bounces out of the bowl, you can bet that the hungry dog will dive for it, totally ignoring the bowl for the beginning of the shot. Enough of these misses and the once ravenous star is sated; then the eating sequence has to be postponed, or the whole commercial reshot with another dog.

Very pregnant, and wearing a black waffle-piqué maternity dress, I showed up at the appointed hour at CBS studios for a Revlon Love Pat commercial. We were still live then, (as opposed to "live on tape" as is often the case today), and so rehearsals and blocking of the commercial began hours before actual air time.

My only shot in this commercial was to stroke a large white Persian cat with my perfectly manicured bejeweled hand, thereby emphasizing the softness and elegance of the makeup in the ad. The large fluffy cat was seated on my lap, nestled on the shelf my pregnant tummy provided. The black piqué of the dress made a perfect backdrop for the shot. It seemed to be an ideal job for me, as I didn't have to do any of the bending and stretching, which were getting tougher as my delivery date drew near. The blocking and rehearsal hours went so smoothly that just stroking a beautiful pussycat on cue seemed an embarrassingly easy way to make money. As the actual show began, somehow the cat sensed the excitement, and as the red light went on for my action cue, she urinated copiously all over me. The black piqué of my dress showed none of this to camera, but the sensation I experienced was unbelievable. Wet warm cat urine was all over me. When the shot was completed the trainer took the cat from me. As I arose, my black piqué maternity dress was plastered to my protruding stomach. I just hated myself. I quickly took a taxi home, removed the dress and threw it down the incinerator.

2110169

ONE HAND WASHES THE OTHER (SOMETIMES)

Most working professional hand models are a joy to work with, and when employed in tandem, we usually entertain each other by relating our latest tales of triumph or torture with the various film directors in town. English hand model Jean Rayner is not only an accurate craftsman, she is one of my best friends. We have spent many a day diapering babies for a disposable-diaper manufacturer, managing to catch up on the latest gossip at the same time. Actually we regard a booking that will involve working together as a cash savings in toll telephone calls.

Occasionally, however, the person you are cast to work with is not so pleasant. I have had to hand sticks of gum or goblets full of liquid to people whose hands were shaking so badly that we couldn't get the shot. This can be because they have been drinking, are very nervous, or have been excessively fatigued by a thoughtless director's insistence that they remain in an uncomfortable position while the cameraman sets his shot, everyone in the agency gets to look through the camera, and four clients request lighting or framing changes.

LIVE TV

Live television commercials, rarely done since the widespread use of video tape, really separated the men from the boys in surviving the effects of excitement. Try rushing from one set to another (sometimes even one studio to another within the time span of a single show), all the while keeping cool enough to pick up a tiny lipstick without showing as much as a flicker of nerves.

My first live commercial was for Kent cigarettes, who sponsored the "$64,000 Challenge." Bob Wright was the announcer, and, on cue, in the middle of his pitch, he was to hand me a lit Kent cigarette. Actually I was about twenty feet away from him in my own setup, with my own camera to cover the closeup of the lit cigarette in my hand, coupled with a "beauty shot" of a package of Kents. The cigarettes for closeups were always lit by prop men who specialized in drawing the exact amount of smoke through the cigarette to produce a perfect ash. The rehearsals went smoothly, and I figured that I was lucky to have little to do but just be there and look good for my first live show.

I was very excited at the prospect of my hands being seen live by millions of people, as this was a tremendously popular show. Actual air time arrived, and about three-quarters of the way through the program, our commercial began. As Wright began his pitch, my hand was poised above the ashtray in full view of my camera. As the red light went on my camera, signifying that we were on the air, I was horrified to see that there was no cigarette in my hand. The prop man had somehow

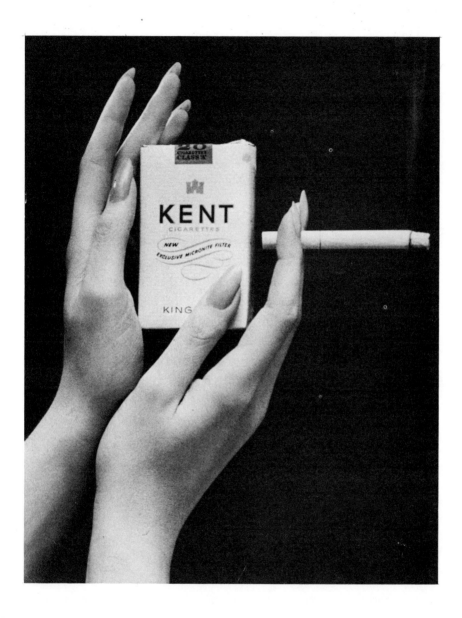

missed his cue to light up. All I could do was stare at the TV monitor showing my bare hand elegantly, but meaninglessly curved over the ashtray. When the show was over, we redid the commercial for the kinescope that would go out to the West Coast. No one seemed very concerned with the goof. The sponsors told me that because my hand was so steady, most viewers probably thought I actually had a cigarette in my hand. It was very lucky my hand never betrayed what my stomach felt at that moment.

THE IMPORTANCE OF BEING
A PROPERTY MAN

Property men or "props," as they are called, can make or break your day. Good ones know how to hollow out a heavy bottle so it will be easier to handle, and to weight one that is too light to place with easy accuracy. They can set up a rig for an arm rest to steady your hand, score the back of a foil packet so that it will pour more easily, and strip the inside of a bottle cap so that it can be removed in one turn. They can hand you the "fresh" product right side up so that you place it on your marks just right. In other words, good prop men can make you look good. A bad prop may, however, not pay attention to the director, not be prepared with enough "product" to cover a sufficient number of takes, and be generally apathetic to your cause. There are very few of these around any more, mainly because I have killed a few myself.

MY NIGHT WITH HAZEL BISHOP

After I had done several live commercials for Revlon, Kent, Lux liquid, Ipana, etcetera, I was booked for two shows on a Saturday night just around Christmas for Hazel Bishop cosmetics. Although I had been warned that these people could be very difficult (as were all cosmetic accounts), I fearlessly, and as it turned out foolishly, considered myself an old hand at the problems of live TV, as well as cosmetic demonstration.

In the commercial I would be wearing a gold lamé glove while picking up and manipulating the swivel feature of a metal lipstick. While the glittery glove looked lovely on camera, it was slippery material and would give little grip.

On the actual day of the show, the lady producer, who had eagerly cast me just two days before, was dissatisfied with me. No one could figure out exactly what the problem was, but it was probably a combination of the extreme pressure of the Christmas commercials and the demanding head of Hazel Bishop, to whom she was directly responsible. Nothing I did pleased her. As we set each shot, she would come bounding out of the TV control room, shrieking "No, no, no. Wrong. Stupid," and proceed to demonstrate to me and all those in the studio how she wished each move of my hands to be. Then she would go back into the control room to watch me try to accomplish what she felt she could do so easily and adeptly. And no sooner did the red light of my camera go on than she would burst out of the control room, each time berating me louder than the time before. Apparently she trusted no one to do these demos but herself and wanted to be the one to do the shots.

And so, after about an hour of agonizing and embarrassing camera rehearsal, she announced that I was fired, and that she would, in fact, do the two shows herself. And so this self ap-pointed wonderwoman was going to be the first producer who also doubled as a hand model. Live yet. And at Christmas.

Because she was at least smart enough to realize that her hands were not cosmetically acceptable to the critical camera eye, she wore the lamé gloves for all three spots. On air she was way off her marks in placing the products down, and when she had to hold the lipstick, she was out of frame entirely! Unfortu-nately I couldn't even gloat, because the fact that she was wear-ing gloves obscured the true identity of the hand model, and everyone not in the studio, including the head of the company, thought it was I who had seriously botched the job. I'm told he forbade "that hand model" to ever work for Hazel Bishop again.

CHORUS GIRL NAILS

When the movie *That's Entertainment* was the hit of the year, Busby Berkeley-style large production numbers were flourishing in TV commercials. The advertising agency for Sally Hansen Hard as Nails Enamel designed their own version, cleverly using nails and fingers as their "chorus girls." A marvelous Art Deco stage was built to scale so that the fingers (in costume) appeared to be dancers as they descended the mirrored platforms and took center stage. A recording was made with an original jingle sung by a spirited chorus of girls. The sounds of tap dancing by what seemed to be a cast of thousands completed the old MGM extravaganza effect.

Three hand models were carefully cast, chosen as much for their coordination and similarity of size of their fingers as for the esthetic qualities of their nails. Each pair of dancing hands that auditioned had to show how well she could step and kick to the music. Getting the job seemed to be a special plum because the shoot was to take at least three days, which is a long booking for a single commercial. We were also told that the novelty of the concept was sure to be the talk of the industry, if not the entire American viewing public. The promise of instant fame as the "Sally Hansen Dancing Fingernails" was known only to the likes of Ruby Keeler.

The characters in Michael Bennett's *A Chorus Line* couldn't have been more pleased with being chosen than Jean Rayner, Pat Tilly and I, as we eagerly reported for fittings for our "costumes" and rehearsals. On the first day of actual shooting, we all arrived joyfully juiced up for "lights, camera and action." Setting up the shot, the director realized that the only way we would be able to "dance" unseen was to suspend us on a platform above the miniature stage. So we all climbed up onto this wooden plank and prepared for the making of our musical. Unfortunately, lying on your stomach on a wooden plank for several hours can become extremely painful. Our arms ached, our backs ached, even our breasts ached from the hard surface, so that we eventually had to inch up and extend over the platform from our waists, putting an incredible strain on our backs.

The first day was tough and uncomfortable, but we were all real troupers and pressed on. They had yet to get a perfect take for rhythm, choreography and camera. On the second day we were experiencing tender skin from lying on the wood for eight hours the previous day, in addition to aching arm and back muscles. By the third day we all agreed that we would gladly pay *them* to get out of this job.

As for our budding celebrity, somewhere during the third day of shooting, the client became disenchanted with the dancing nails concept as a major sales thrust in the cosmetics market and claimed he had never okayed the costs of the sets, costumes and recording. Although the ad agency thought the finished commercial was the best work it had ever produced, the spot was never aired once. Alas, fame on the Great White Way is so fleeting.

ARE YOUR HANDS INSURED?

The first time somebody asked me if my hands were insured was in December 1958. I remember it well. "Of course not." How silly. How indulgent! I thought. My former husband was a serious skier, and we were planning a holiday on the Vermont slopes. After careful consideration, I decided that skiing was much too dangerous a sport for me. In an effort to be a good little wife and have my own cold-weather sport, I took up ice skating. I bought special expensive skates, took special expensive lessons, and of course, bought special expensive little outfits. My husband dropped me off at the local rink in Stowe, on his way to Mount Mansfield for a day of skiing. The temperature in Vermont was so cold that there were pressure cracks in the ice at the rink. Being the basically careful person that I am, I just performed very slow movements, perfecting my figure eights and threes, smug that I had taken all the sensible precautions and wasn't participating in the more hazardous sport of skiing. Suddenly, in an accident that could happen in my own living room, I turned the wrong way, my skate caught an edge, lodged itself in a pressure crack, and I fell, breaking the fall with my wrist. And that's not all I broke. My wrist was broken—only a hairline fracture, but broken. While I was spending the rest of my vacation in a cast, Revlon called to book me for their show the following week. I said, "I don't know how to tell you this, but I broke my wrist." Typically, the Revlon spokesman said, "But you couldn't have!" I don't know whose power did the healing, but the cast was off and I was back working for Revlon in less than four weeks.

AGENTS

Talent agent Martha Robertson has probably booked more hand commercials than anyone in the world. She refers to hand modeling as the most professional part of the business. She explained that hand models must show the least ego. Because the successful ones work more actual filming days than on-camera talent (exclusivity is not an employment factor if you aren't recognizable), lapses in promptness, cooperation and steadiness are more obvious. Like the new pretty face in town, a perfectly beautiful or masculine pair of hands won't last long in the business if it isn't accompanied by the skills and behavior of the pro.

Robertson told me that the most bizarre request ever made of her by a client was when an ad agency needed an arthritic hand model for Bufferin. "Now, how can a hand model have arthritis and still work?" she pondered. In addition, the agency requested that the model to be booked have arthritis in the third finger, right hand (in order to comply with the requirements of the story board). Absurd as the request was, she toiled away and got as good a match as she could: a woman who had, in fact, done hand modeling, and now suffered from arthritis. The only compromise was that the arthritis was in her third finger, left hand. Needless to say, the agency booked the model, flopped the required image, and Robertson became the fairhaired girl of hand bookers, having produced a minor casting miracle.

AT HOME WITH KENT CIGARETTES

Sets and setups for commercials can be as simple as a tabletop or as elaborate as the elegant two-room "apartment" complete with fine paintings and Baccarat crystal. Director Mike Cimino (who many years later was to make the Academy Award-winning *The Deer Hunter*) was so thorough in his preparation for a certain Kent commercial that he created a whole history and situation for his characters. The husband, who was featured on camera, already successful (as evidenced by this grand home), had just been given a large promotion which could mean impressive changes in his life. He and his wife are celebrating at dinner. She is happy, but knows that their life will never be the same, never as close. And so a bittersweet note also pervades the evening. We spent two days toasting with wine, touching hands and dancing. "Days of Wine and Roses" played in the background. The mood was maintained so completely that at the end of the filming, I felt that I had actually lived in that apartment. And to this day, when I hear that song, a wave of nostalgia comes over me.

The whole commercial was thirty seconds long in its final cut.

It was shown once, on the Ed Sullivan show.

TRYING NOT TO BITE
THE HAND THAT FEEDS YOU

Because of my unique position of doing the hands for many competitors, I am very selective about involving myself in "tests" where an endorsement is concerned. Some years ago, while I was doing one or two shows a week for Revlon, I was asked to participate in a Jergens Lotion test. In past years, after extensive research, the Jergens test situation was repeated in a hotel room in New York city with models who could be used in photography and commercials. Both hands were soaked three times a day in hot soapy water, and Jergens applied to only one hand. Hopefully the resulting difference would be dramatic enough to show up on a film. And it always was. The extreme cold temperatures of a January day accelerated the reddening effect of the "bad" hand, which many of us actually kept more exposed than the other, being eager to be chosen for the actual campaign. This was before the heavier government restrictions that were to come later, and no one cared much because there was no competing product involved.

This time, however, we were instructed to apply a Brand X on the bad hand before soaking, and Jergens afterward. We were all busy applying lots of Jergens in between soaks (as we were given a supply to take home with us for overnight applications), and, as before, all making sure that the bad hand got plenty of exposure to the cold weather. As the last "legally required" soak was completed, we were given affidavits to sign, before a chosen few would be taxied over to the photographer's studio. As all the other girls happily signed away, I read the actual document and was concerned to find that it clearly stated that "at no time did I apply Jergens lotion without an equal application of Brand X."

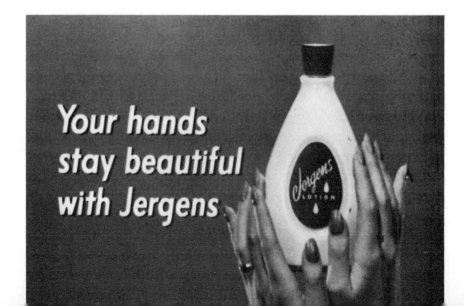

Since we had never been so instructed (actually we never received any Brand X for application away from the testing site), I inquired as to the identity of Brand X. I was casually told that Brand X was, in fact, Revlon's Silicare Lotion, and that they were hoping to provoke Revlon into a lawsuit with their "findings." I wouldn't sign, as it was not only "biting the hand that fed me" at least twice a week, but it also wasn't true. They were furious, as I was apparently first choice for the campaign. But falsely testifying in a suit against Revlon, or anyone else, was not exactly what I needed to further my career.

CATCH A FALLING STAR

One TV star, known more for her hairdo than her acting ability, insisted that my hands duplicate hers as closely as possible for the product shots of a commercial she was pitching. She not only rejected the polish the director had chosen for its photogenic quality, but she also wanted my skin made up to be as dark as hers. She chose the nail color, the length of my nails and even the shape of my nails. I had to devise a special combination of polishes to duplicate exactly what her nails looked like "bare." After I had produced a near-perfect "match," the director asked me if I could just take my nails down "a pfuffky more." I answered that "short of breaking one and biting two, this was as close a match as we were going to get!"

BEHIND THE SCENES

People usually assume a day's work on a TV set is glamorous, but behind the scenes is another story. For one thing, this work is generally uncomfortably hot. The shots are not lit with your comfort in mind. The product is the star and you have to position yourself sandwiched in between the lights, which are sometimes so strong that you can actually feel your hair burning.

Some directors who specialize in tabletop, or product, shots routinely supply the hand model with an aluminum "hat" for protection.

Also hand models often have to wear the clothes worn by the principal of the commercial. This can sometimes mean being draped in a top many times too small for you, revealing all too much flesh from the back view. The worst indignity, however, is being told to don a dress that is dripping wet with someone else's perspiration after an unusually long or arduous filming. It doesn't happen often, but when it does it feels like a good enough reason to leave the business.

Sometimes the demands of a commercial are simply too intimate for comfort. When Revlon was promoting gold nail enamel, the shades they produced did not read "gold" enough for camera, so they provided me with real gold paint for the actual commercial. The problem was that everyone's nails excrete minute amounts of natural oils, and so the gold paint never really dried. It would be necessary to apply the gold paint to my nails around 2 P.M. in time for the on-camera rehearsals. However, show time wasn't until nine o'clock. Head stylist Pat Reynolds, whose job it was to coordinate the whole look of the commercial, attended to every detail with martial dedication. This meant that if I had to go to the bathroom, she would have to accompany me to the ladies' room to negotiate my girdle and stockings as the slightest friction would have caused the gold paint to "curdle." I was very grateful for the eventual passing of my career as Revlon's personal "Gold Finger."

Frequently the product shots you are hired to do are the very chores that will enable you to make enough money to ensure that you never have to do them at home. As I was wiping off the most disgusting baked-on grease from the inside of an oven, I thought that I should be the one to ask, "What's a nice girl like you doing in a place like this?" (At least the on-camera actress is getting residuals each time the commercial is shown. That's what *she's* doing there!)

I have probably done enough dishes, pots and laundry to

feed and clothe the whole United States Army. In one week I cleaned bathrooms for Pine-Sol, Comet and Sani-Flush. Coincidentally, the same cameraman was on all three jobs. As he directed me as to which portion of the "bathroom bowl" (TV jargon for "toilet") should frame the product I was holding, I realized this all had a familiar ring to it—and looked up at him and said, "Freddie, we have got to stop meeting like this!"

DEFINITELY OUT OF HAND

I reluctantly accepted a booking for a third reshot on a shoe-polish commercial. I was leaving early in the morning on vacation and I requested, and got, a promise of release by 10 P.M. Ten o'clock came and went, as we continued with new shots, not previously discussed, being added to the agenda. As we went into the wee small hours, the nervous clients and the paranoid producer ignored my request to leave. At 2 A.M., a white nurse's shoe was produced for me to put on. I was to wear the shoe while polishing it for camera. Not only is this hard on the back, but the big problem was that the shoe was a 5B and I wear an 8½ AAA. When I complained that the shoe didn't fit, the agency man shot back with "That's what you told us your size was," thus trying to protect himself. I answered that even if I wanted to lie about my shoe size, who would believe me? All anyone had to do was look at my long skinny foot to know I couldn't wear a size 5B. Again I asked to leave, as it was way past my promised release time. At that moment a member of the staff locked the doors of the studio and told me, "You will finish the shot or I will tell the union that you walked out. It will be your word against ours." I was frightened not only by their numbers, but also by their clout. Would you believe that I actually squeezed my foot into the shoe for the shot? It was excruciating, but I would have done anything short of suicide to get out of the studio that night. And, of course, I was short-changed on the payment.

The Language

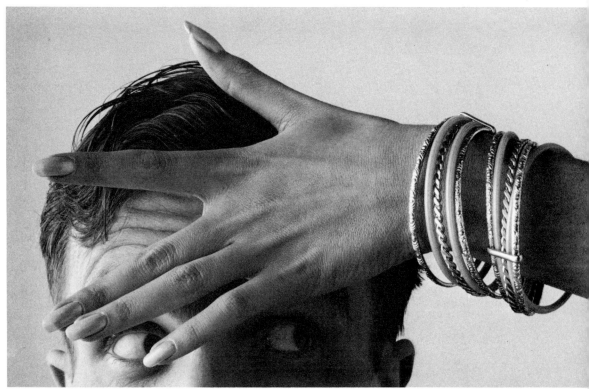

STANLEY JOHNSON

of Hands

Rituals and Signals

ALTHOUGH THE PARLOR GAME charades points up the difficulties of silent communication, hand gestures often speak louder than words, to paraphrase an old saying.

A simple hand gesture from the referee of a sports event, or from a traffic cop, or a prelate's hand raised in blessing, or the affectionate touch from a loved one can elicit enormous emotional response or communicate more than the most eloquent prose. Even TV directors and recording-sound engineers all have special hand languages that make possible the silent communication required by their jobs.

A person's spontaneous gestures may provide us with more information about him than his words. Consider the automatic social labeling of a "boardinghouse reach." The meaning of conscious and unconscious hand signals varies widely from one culture to another; Occidental viewers of the Japanese Kabuki theater, for example, often miss the intended meaning of many of the gestures used.

During the Kefauver Committee hearings on crime in our society, gangland chieftain Frank Costello's hands became famous when he refused to allow his face to be televised and only his hands were visible on TV.

While the value of character study through graphology (personality reading through handwriting analysis) and palmistry (personality reading through study of the shape and lines of the hand), is considered by many to be limited, elements of these two "sciences" are gradually becoming accepted tools in medical diagnoses of certain diseases.

THE HANDSHAKE

Campaigning politicians, who shake more hands than anyone, have found that the handshake creates the strongest possible bond with the greatest number of people in the least amount of time. The handshake was originally a greeting among males born out of mutual distrust. When men carried swords, an extended right hand meant you were not reaching for a weapon.

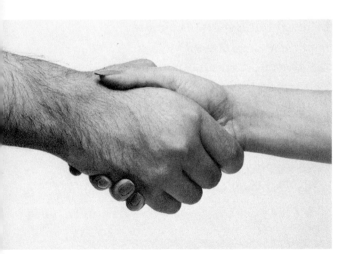

The traditional handshake

The outstretched hand showed that you were not concealing anything. As women were included in this ritual, etiquette demanded that the woman extend her hand first. Proper handshaking protocol varies from culture to culture, and even in the United States it is often unclear as to whether one is to shake in the traditional manner or perform the newer "soul, hippie, what's happenin' " handshake (thumbs locked and doubled fists) often expected by rock musicians, athletes and a large proportion of the population under thirty years of age.

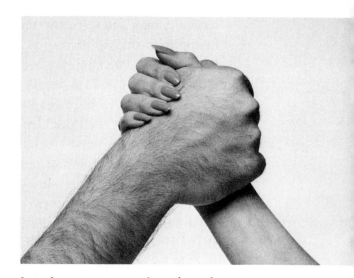

The "soul," "hippie," or "what's happenin' " handshake

This "soul" shake can take place between two close friends as well as strangers, whereas the traditional handshake, if it appears without any accompanying gestures, usually signifies a lack of intimacy between the two participants. How far one extends his hand from his body during the shake is actually evidence of the desired distance he is putting between himself and the person to whom he is offering his hand. Thrusting your hand far in front of you keeps the person at arm's length.

When greeted by an overly strong handshake you are being told by the person that they want you to notice their directness and sincerity. If the palm portion of the hand you are grabbing feels strong and resilient, this is probably a true character trait. If the handshake is not only strong, but also overlong, the person is making an attempt to make special contact, usually of a sexual nature. You can actually tell a little about the sexuality of the person during the initial handshake by noting if he seems to enjoy the tactile contact, feel of skin, and seems anxious to prolong the physical contact. Also note whether or not he is sensitive to your response, or is being insistently aggressive. If you subtly pull away, and he hangs on, watch out! He will demand his own way. A weak and flabby handshake reveals disinterest. The person lacks vitality in general, or at least where you are concerned. If the palm is also soft, be warned that the person is basically lazy and self-centered. You will have to do all the work in the relationship. If you go to shake a person's hand, and his hand retreats the slightest bit, he is either insincere or has been hurt. He doesn't want to say "Hello." If, conversely, you pull back, you will literally get hurt, because the other person will then grab you at the knuckles.

Grabbing the person's right hand with both hands is another gesture of warmth, sometimes used to plead with or convince the other person to do something. Desmond Morris correlates the progression of involvement of the left hand and arm in a right-handed shake with the degree of intimacy the two people share. He charts the progression from the singlehanded shake to the shake with the left-handed squeeze, followed by touching the right arm, the shoulder reach, and finally the handshake where the hand circles the shoulders in a one arm embrace, which demonstrates the affectionate familiarity.

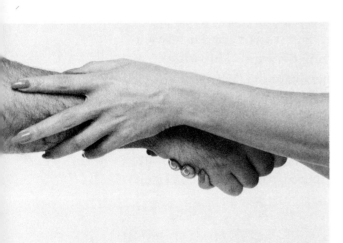

The intimate handshake

THE ROYAL TOUCH

Members of royalty, pontiffs and prophets are considered by many to be the middlemen between God and ordinary mortals. Because they are thought to be invested with superhuman powers, either by virtue of their birth, commitment or knowledge, they are believed by some to act as a perfect channel for transmitting divine vibrations to the masses.

HAND-KISSING

Hand-kissing has its roots in early religious ritual, as it evolved from the custom of kissing the papal ring to show devout honor and respect. During the middle ages, knights would express their homage to a lady by kissing her hand, and to this day, it is considered to be a gallant and continental custom. Although considered an act of politeness in Central Europe, hand-kissing in Spain and Italy is practiced only between close relatives.

CARRYING THE BRIDE
OVER THE THRESHOLD

This custom might be a behavioral extension of sitting on a parent's or boy friend's lap—a combination of adolescent sexuality and infantile cuddling. It also enacts the masculine gesture of literally "taking" the bride into his own territory.

THE MARRIAGE RING FINGER

It was once believed that the shortest vein or artery to the heart was from the fourth finger of the left hand. This may have accounted for the ritualistic use of this finger for placement of the wedding ring. A more sensible explanation is that the left hand is more convenient for wearing jewelry, as most people are right-handed. Also, the fourth finger is the only finger that cannot be extended alone and is therefore protected by the others. *Note:* Some palmists believe that a very prominent mount under the ring finger indicates a vulnerability to heart disease.

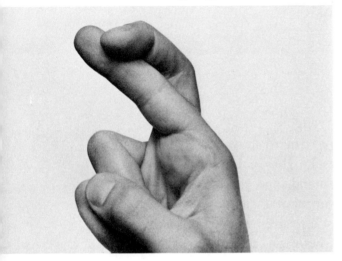

Here's hoping

CROSSING THE FINGERS

Crossing the fingers is actually making a sign of the cross and is an ancient Christian protective device, like crossing oneself. It is a method of wishing oneself or another good luck, as well as exonerating oneself from the dire consequences of a lie. Knocking on wood after announcing some enormous good fortune is another way of placating the gods.

SHAKING YOUR OWN HANDS
ABOVE YOUR HEAD

Shaking your own hands above your head is used as a sign of triumph, especially by professional fighters. The person is taking center stage and announcing "Cheers for me" (or us). He is augmenting his body height as well as leaving his chest unprotected to demonstrate his invincibility.

OK SIGN

The circle formed by the thumb and forefinger symbolizes perfection in America as well as in many cultures throughout the world. Desmond Morris notes, however, that in Japan, the circle means money (resembling the shape of a coin), while in some parts of France it is the symbol for zero, nothing, worthlessness. And in Malta, Sardinia and Greece, it is an obscene insult.

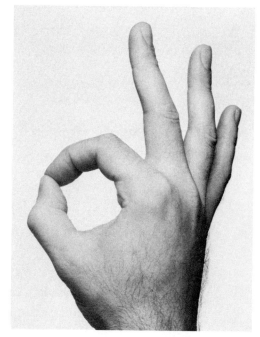

A-OK

THUMBS UP OR THUMBS DOWN

Thumbs up or thumbs down tells the outcome or decision on something or someone. It is possibly derived from the practice of spectators at Roman gladiator contests, who, by the position

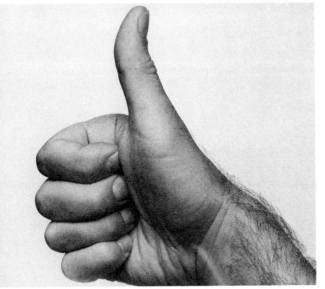

Thumbs up

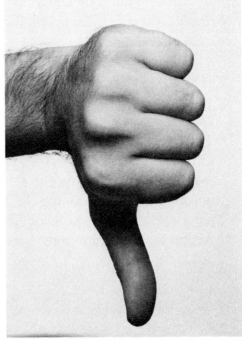

Thumbs down

of their thumbs, signaled the victor whether or not to kill his defeated opponent.

THE PEACE SIGN

Holding the index and second fingers up to form a V is the same as the V for victory sign used by Winston Churchill during World War II. Although the sign is usually done with the palm facing out, if the V is formed with the palm toward the gesturer, the signal has an obscene meaning in many parts of the world.

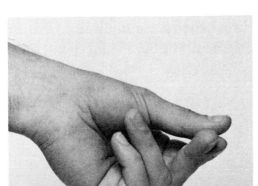

Gimme some

RUBBING THE THUMB AND FOREFINGER TOGETHER

Rubbing the thumb and forefinger together is a signal to pay up, or a communication that money is coming.

LEFT-HANDEDNESS

Left-handed people are treated like second-class citizens in this right-handed world. Tools, instruments and cars are made for the right-handed. All people are expected to salute, as well as shake hands, with the right hand. And eating side by side with a left-handed person can be inconvenient if you are not placed correctly. Furthermore, left-handed terms are mainly derogatory. The "left-handed compliment" is lacking graciousness. *Gauche,* the French word for "left," is used in English to describe a clumsy or awkward action. "Sinister" is derived from the Latin word for "left-handed."

Among identical twins—those who develop from the same ovum—usually one is left-handed, as if each were a mirror image of the other. It has been theorized that some of the left-handed people of the world represent a twin whose sister or brother did not survive the gestation period in the womb.

Among the famous artists who were lefthanded were Michelangelo and Holbein.

THE SINISTER SIDE OF TENNIS

Left-handed tennis champion Rosco Tanner: "Being left-handed used to be an advantage in tennis, but now as many as 35 to 40 percent of the leading players are left-handed, so it no longer gives me an edge."

Gestures

TRYING NOT TO "TIP YOUR HAND"

All gestures have two purposes: to help discharge tension and to communicate or punctuate conversation. (God knows, I don't think I could hold a conversation with hands behind my back!) Sometimes the hand gesture is contradictory to what the speaker is verbalizing. Or occasionally the gesture is totally in keeping with what the person is saying, but is so out of proportion to the evident emotional investment of the speaker, that it appears unbelievable or phony. This phenomenon is frequently seen in politicians professionally trained in "image-making." Mimic David Frye is a master at picking up these gestures and exaggerating them further, rendering the politician he's portraying hilariously absurd, rather than presenting the zealously earnest picture that is, of course, the conscious intention of the speaker.

HAND-TO-HEAD GESTURES

All gestures are learned, conscious or unconscious, and so are culturally determined. Our conscious, as well as unconcious, signal for "Halt!" (pushing away with one or both palms extended) is ironically the same as the Nazi salute. The learning process starts in early infancy when the baby explores his face and mouth. Putting his fingers in his mouth is pleasurable, as it satisfies his need to suck as well as simulating the action of feeding. As adults we often do the same sort of hand-to-mouth action when we are in need of assistance, reassurance or inspiration. Most ex-smokers will attest to the difficulty of giving up this infantile addiction.

While an adult will occasionally resort to putting a finger in his mouth while contemplating a problem, the accepted mature derivative behavior is more apt to take the form of rubbing the chin, or nose (puzzlement), scratching the head or chin, stroking the nose with the index finger, placing the two index fingers by the sides of the mouth, or cupping the chin as in Rodin's "The Thinker." Some of these "thinking" gestures express doubt. The hand to the eye or temple says "I don't know. I'll have to think about that. I don't trust that." These actions give us the space of infantile safety in which to ponder a question. The hand to the forehead, sometimes shadowing the eyes, is a more sophisticated form of shutting out external stimuli in order to tap one's inner mental resources. This pose is sometimes assumed in prayer or meditation for communication with higher sources. Show biz "psychics" often use this gesture to convince the audience that they are in touch with unspoken information. In his portrayal of "The Great Karnak" TV MC Johnny Carson uses this gesture as an absurd caricature to indicate that he is being "divinely inspired" with the correct answer.

HAND-TO-HEAD GESTURES
SHOWING EMBARRASSMENT

Covering the mouth or the whole profile with the hand serves to protect yourself from your own unspoken words and is a reaction to the fear of self exposure. We also cover our eyes when we are ashamed, in an attempt to shut out the rest of the world from our behavior.

SURPRISE OR SHOCK

More rapid hand-to-head movements signify recognition or surprise. Slapping the forehead says, "Oh, my God, I forgot to do that," while slapping one or both hands to the cheeks expresses disbelief at receiving shockingly good (or bad) information. This is sometimes known as the "Oh, no" or "Holy shit" gesture.

THE SELF-SLAP

This is a basically hostile act turned toward oneself, saying "Pay attention, dummy." When we are in a fit of laughter, we will

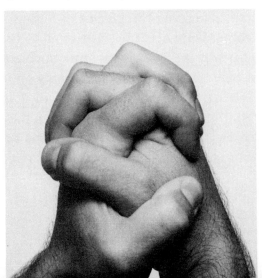

Death grip

occasionally slap our sides, or knees, as if the slap will bring the body back under control. Sometimes the person will use the self-slap to prove that he is enjoying another person's humor more than is actually the case.

HOW YOU CARRY YOUR HANDS

You can tell a lot about a person's disposition without his saying a word. A person who carries his arms folded in front of his chest is extremely self-protective and is saying, "Dare me" or "You can't get at me." It is a stance reminiscent of defiance of one's parents. Similarly, hands on the hips is the pose of the bully who feels confident of his strength in a situation. He is saying, "Just try it." A person seated with hands clasped behind his head, leaning back on his chair, displays the ultimate self-confidence and independence. If this position is assumed in a group gathering or meeting, he sets himself apart as the one who has to be convinced by the others. His pose says, "I am strong enough to be open to all you have to say, but I alone will be the final judge of the value of what you say."

TIGHTLY LOCKED FINGERS

Tightly locked fingers are a way of holding oneself together. Most of us use some method of "holding on" in unfamiliar situations. We reach for Mommy when we are unsure as babies, and now we seek to reduce the tension by pulling at our fingers, rings, tie, wringing our hands, or even digging our fingernails into the palms or nail bed. Our hands can hover around our necks in a symbolic effort to "save our necks." Women sometimes try to disguise this hand-to-neck movement as a careless sweep of the hair. (This can also be a seductive gesture if stroking the hair is a substitute for stroking the shoulders or breasts.) Discomfort can be expressed as subtly as the light tapping of a finger, signifying impatience, or as intensely as gripping on to the arms of a chair in order to "hold on for dear life."

HANDS IN THE POCKETS

Keeping the hands in the pockets or behind the back is usually the action of someone who has something to hide. It can also be interpreted as a sign of laziness, or an unwillingness to pitch in (or shell out). Another version of this hand position signifies non-involvement. It then becomes a "cool" gesture, as exemplified by the sophistication of Fred Astaire dancing entire musical numbers with his hands in his pockets.

PALMS

The palms thrust out in front of the speaker say "Now, wait a minute, back off. I'm protecting my space. You've gone about as far as you can go with me." Holding the palms upward implies the speaker is begging for something from the listener. Opening the palms to the speaker and then rotating them says, "It doesn't matter. Either way is OK," as in the German *Machts Nichts.* The palms reverse to a downward position if the conversation becomes too heated, in an effort to "lower the flame." The two

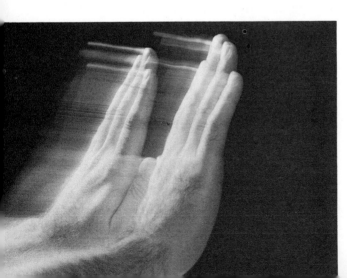

Back off

palms facing each other is an effort to "box in" the speaker's thoughts. He is attempting to put everything both of you are saying together in order to view it as a whole. It is a plea to "be reasonable," and so is conciliatory.

The hand placed with the palm touching the heart is protective, or a signal of the truth, as in "I swear to God." Often a person asking for a loan will make this gesture to show his honesty and to protect himself from possible rejection. This hand-on-the-heart gesture is also used, often in an exaggerated form (and rarely with the proper effectiveness), by trained politicians.

RUBBING THE HANDS TOGETHER

Rubbing the hands together signifies satisfaction or anticipation, and says "Oh, goody. I can't wait to get my hands on you (or it)." Beware of buying from a vendor who does this, as it can be evidence of a Uriah Heap syndrome.

SYMBOLIC HAND-WASHING

Symbolic hand-washing is done by wiping each palm with the palm of the other hand to free it of any last traces of the situation one wants to be finished with. This gesture symbolizes the close of a cycle, saying, "That's the end of that."

HOSTILE GESTURES

Shaking a fist, rubbing the nose, or holding an open palm up, as if to warn a child of a forthcoming spanking, are all gestures that

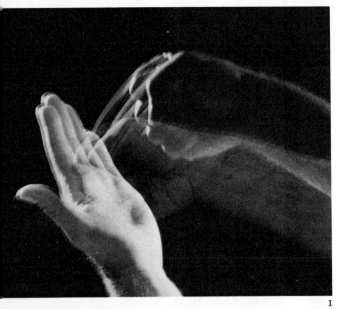

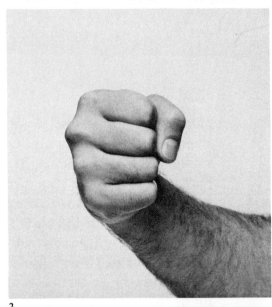

1 2

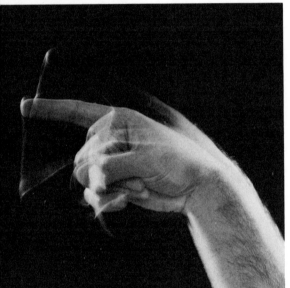

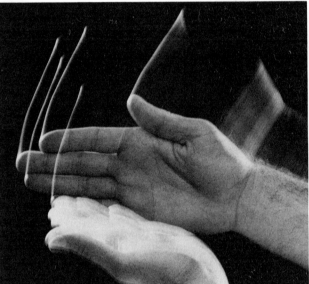

3 4

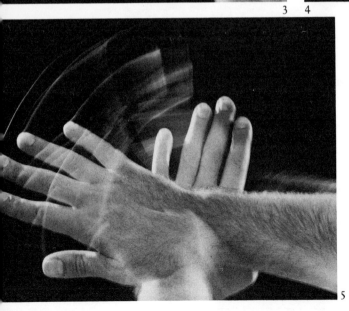

5

1. A fist smacked into the palm says "I've been had," or "I knew it all the time!"

2. Shaking a fist

3. A "no-no"

4. Hand chop

5. The "no way"

complete a conversation wordlessly. They all say "Back off."

A raised index finger can be a silent attempt to dominate by warning that you are already armed. When used together with words, it can be a subtle aid in accentuating a point. But if the speaker actually touches the other person with his index finger he is, in effect, dealing a blow. The fingernail is seen here as an extension of the hand, and as a potential weapon. Bitten nails are often a sign of repressed hostility, so if the speaker's are bitten, he will likely be highly critical, especially of himself. And he has literally "cut off his own weapons."

A vertically held hand comes down forcefully on the other hand, which is held horizontally with the palm up. It signifies the speaker's desire to cut through the confusion and find a solution, even if it means imposing his ideas on you. The slashing of the hand is like an ax, ready to cut you off. The "no way" is similar to the hand chop, but here both hands are used to deny or reject the other person's position or information. He is cutting his way through what he perceives to be hostile behavior and attempts to stop the opposition by striking it away with both hands. The verbal equivalent would be "Clear the decks." Politicians often train themselves to use chops, table pounding and clenched fists not only to emphasize their stand on issues, but also to show their constituency that they are willing to fight for them.

AFFECTIONATE GESTURES: WALKING HAND IN HAND

As the infant learns to walk, he reaches for a hand to support him. We hold on to older children to protect them in crowds or where there is traffic. My children were so conditioned to this safety procedure that as one foot left the curb, the hand nearest me would reach up for mine, almost a reflex action. Children will skip along swinging each other by the hand as a sign of

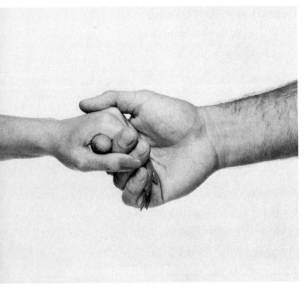

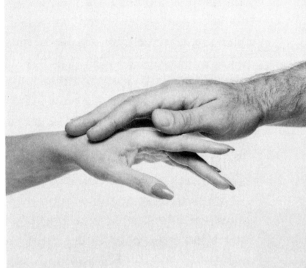

Hand in hand   The pat

friendship, as well as hold on to the shoulders of their buddies. Until adolescence these contacts commonly take place between members of the same sex. At puberty these gestures become sexual and are usually confined to the opposite sex. The female occasionally hooks her arm through that of the male, indicating that he is guide and protector; this gesture is a public display of affection. When an arm is offered in aid to an elderly or frail person, it has no sexual or emotional significance, but is just a gesture of doing a good turn.

Desmond Morris, zoologist and noted author of *The Naked Ape* and *Gestures,* notes that touching someone's head is far more intimate than touching his arm. But when inappropriate, it can be alarming, and may elicit prompt defensive retaliation. It is a gesture usually made between lovers, the closest of friends, or loving parents. The "pat" is described by Morris as a "miniature embrace by the hand alone." A pat can convey a greeting, one's congratulations, or comfort, love or friendship. Children can be patted on most any part of their bodies, whereas adults' pats are confined to the hand, arm, shoulder or back. If, however, an adult is patted on the head, buttocks, thighs or knees, a sexual or condescending note is in evidence.

THE HUG

Children are hugged all the time, whether they want it or not. It sort of comes with the job. Young lovers will often hug in public. Adults, however, usually confine hugs to farewells, reunions or times of grief. Hugging as a sexual posture between adults usually takes place in private.

THE WAVE

The wave is a gesture that simulates touch when two parties are separated by distance. A wave "Hello" can be used to get the attention of the other, whereas a wave "Goodbye" is a last or final effort to sustain the physical or emotional tie while actually moving apart. All babies are taught to wave "Bye-bye" to their parents and others. Waving goodbye to intimates can sometimes evoke intense feelings of sadness and separation in adults.

THROWING A KISS

This is a more obvious effort to sustain an emotional tie with the other person while moving apart. Although the wave can be a casual gesture between acquaintances, throwing a kiss implies intimacy. An actress may blow kisses to imply that intimacy exists between her and her public.

TICKLING

Tickling is the light but purposeful touching of another's body that elicits an extremely sensitive response, usually laughter. It is often sexual, and can be an effective controlling device, putting the victim in a bondage-like situation. Children are especially prey to this type of disguised hostility or sexuality either by grownups or groups of their peers.

THE AFFECTIONATE ATTACK

Hair ruffling, arm punches, squeezes and nudges are all seemingly aggressive actions which can be performed without hurting the recipient and take place mostly between males. They provide a socially acceptable opportunity for members of the same sex to touch. These gestures have a sexual undertone when the adolescent tomboy engages in "buddy-buddy" scrapping with a boy. The tomboy works off her hostility toward the male, meanwhile satisfying her less obvious sexual desires for physical contact.

Like tickling, Children are often subjected to overzealous adults who abuse this privilege.

HOW THE SEXUAL TOUCHDOWN
IS SCORED

The cocktail party and the singles bar vie as the mecca of the sexual hand signal. Here the sexual hand signal is as explicit as any verbal exchange between the two people. Some male non-touching sexual hand signals are adjusting the tie, readjusting the clothes (especially pants) and combing or fixing the hair. The man can also hook his thumbs into his belt, pointing his fingers in the direction of his genitals. John Travolta's character Barberino in the TV show "Welcome Back Kotter" used all of these signals to tell the audience that no matter what the predicament of the particular episode he was involved in, his character was always on the make.

Typical female nontouching signals are adjusting the clothes, especially skirt, shoe, or stockings at the ankles. The woman may stroke her thighs as she talks, or she may touch her chest with her fingers pointed down toward her breast.

A male will usually not touch a woman first, except for a handshake, which usually takes place in a party situation when two people are more-or-less formally introduced, and is not a prerequisite to making sexual contact. However, while carrying on a verbal exchange, he can protect his territory with the female by using his arm to block intruding males.

The female makes the first move to touch the male, often by requesting assistance, as in asking for a light for her cigarette. She can then guide his hand with hers. This then gives him permission to move in and touch hands. Julius Fast in his book *Body Language* makes the point that while the male is usually the aggressor in taking the female's hand, he then has to wait for her response of finger pressure before he can interwine his fingers with hers. The next move is the male's arm encircling her shoulders, approaching the breast from the other side and pressing the sides of their bodies together. All of these gestures can occur during conversations no more sexual than the current real estate situation. Once, at a friend's party, the signals between a newly introduced man and myself went so smoothly that several hours later, while discussing the various legal details of his recent divorce, I realized that he was gently squeezing the outside of my thigh. And I hardly noticed because our hand and touch signals had been so thoroughly acknowledged and responded to that it seemed as if we had been intimate a thousand times.

UNDERHANDED SEXUAL SIGNALS

Gestures are sometimes made confidentially by one male to another in order to comment on the sexual attractiveness of a female. If he brings his fingers to his lips and simulates a kiss, he is saying that he finds her to be a delicious dish. Twirling a real or imaginary mustache says the same thing but adds an intention to pursue. Outlining the curve of her waist in the air with his hands signifies that he finds her shapely. Further, cupping his hands under his chest lightly bouncing imaginary breasts notes that she is extremely well endowed or "built." As early as junior high school, if a boy made a circle with the thumb and index finger and inserted the middle finger of the other hand into the circle, he was telling his friends exactly what he wished to do with the female having the attributes noted above. If, however, he picked up the hand belonging to the female who inspired these gestures, and stroked the inside of her palm with his finger, he was clearly communicating to her what his intention was, and risked getting his hand slapped in response to this brazen gesture.

INSULTING GESTURES

Reinforcing the axiom "Actions speak louder than words," a person can use gestures stronger than any verbal taunt to demean another. Children show disrespect by flapping their hands at the sides of their heads, simulating donkey ears. Another derisive gesture children are fond of is thumbing the nose. The schoolyard sign for "Shame on you" is stroking one index finger with the other.

Touching the index finger to the thumb rapidly several times infers that the person being derided is running off at the mouth and his words have no valuable thought behind them. Tapping the temple or rotating the index finger in the temple area says, "You're crazy!" or "You have a screw loose." A limp wrist questions the sexual preference of the male (Italians sometimes express this by touching the ear, suggesting that the man would prefer to wear earrings in private).

When we have had more than enough of a person or situation, we place the hand vertically, with the palm down, at the neck, as if to say, "Any more of this will cause me to vomit." Italians turn this gesture back onto the other person by deliberately stroking from the throat to the chin with four fingers of the hand (palm down), thus saying, "What are you going to do about it?"

Horns made by fingers held to both sides of the head symbolize the cuckhold. It says either that the person is impotent or too stupid to know what's going on with his own wife.

The V, made by holding the index and middle fingers up, popularized by Winston Churchill, says "Peace" or "Victory" when the palm is facing the person signaled. If, however, the back of the hand is away from the signaler, the intent is insulting, and is the equivalent of extending the middle finger in the air.

The "fig" is formed by placing the thumb through the index and middle fingers, while the hand forms a fist. The symbol of this gesture is thought to represent the genitals of the male inserted into the female, and, if viewed as such, is taken as an

Victory   #!*%#!

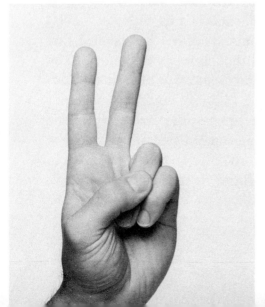

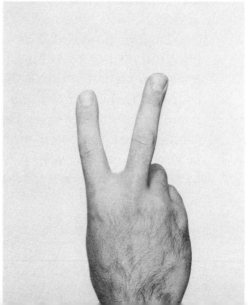

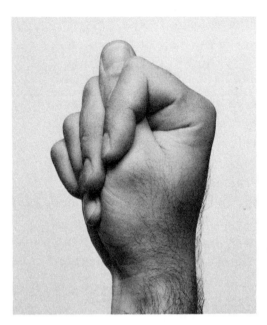

The "fig"

insult. The same gesture, however, is reproduced in the form of jewelry worn for fertility or good luck. Speculation about the origin of the use of the "fig" suggests that it protects the wearer from the evil eye by distracting the attention of the Devil with a pornographic symbol.

The teeth flick is performed by knuckling all but the thumb, while the thumbnail is flicked from behind the front upper teeth toward the person to be insulted. It is Italian in derivation and says, "Go to Hell" or "Get lost." Shakespeare, in *Romeo and Juliet,* makes much of this as an insult, using it as the stimulus for a street fight between Sampson and Abram, in which one says "Do you bite your thumb at us, Sir?"

The "forearm jerk," as Desmond Morris has labeled this universal insult, is phallic, and although it can be performed by either sex, is mainly male. Rather than a simulation of intercourse, it is thought to symbolize an anal assault (although not homosexual). Since street clout equates the size of the male genitalia with the power of the person, a fisted arm is taken to be a much stronger weapon than the middle finger, and so is to be considered the Big Daddy of all the obscene gestures.

THE FINGER

Roger Maris "gave the finger" to the TV camera after hitting a home run, causing a great deal of controversy in sports circles. The most notorious use of this obscene gesture was undoubtedly the night most of America saw comedian Jackie Mason end a mushrooming TV career when he "gave the finger" to the floor director on the Ed Sullivan Show who was giving him the (hand) signal to speed up or end his monologue earlier than Mason thought appropriate. The floor director held up his index finger, which is the sign for "one minute left," and Mason showed his annoyance at being cut short by extending his middle finger, live, on TV, to the largest viewing audience in America at the time.

THE HAND WE CHOOSE TO GESTURE WITH

The right hand is dominated by the left side of the brain, which is responsible for the exercise of thought and conscious activity. Therefore, people who gesture with the right hand are thought to be logical, controlled and well organized. The left hand is dominated by the right side of the brain, which is concerned with instinct, emotions and unconscious desires. People who habitually gesture with the left hand, therefore, tend to be creative and imaginative. It is noted that many show people (who are likely to be creative and imaginative) use their left hands to gesture with.

CULTURAL DIFFERENCES

The amount of gesturing that accompanies conversation is directly in proportion to a person's distance from the Anglo-Saxon model in our society. Immigrants who live in ghettos are more likely to talk with their hands than their American-born second- or third-generation relatives. Often these gestures that are learned in early childhood disappear as the person's vistas change, and they resurface only when he returns to the family group, as on a visit to the old neighborhood, at weddings, confirmations or funerals.

While in the English-speaking world to talk with one's hands is a sign of poor breeding, for Arabs of all social levels gestures are an indispensable part of any conversation. An anthropologist has catalogued no fewer than 247 gestures used by Arabs, the majority of these being obscene. In Jordan and three other Arab countries, to flick the right thumbnail against the front teeth means the gesturer has no money, or only a little, whereas the Italian version of this signal is an obscene expression of anger. Bedouins touch their noses three times to show friendship. In Libya, men twist the tips of their forefingers into their cheeks when speaking to beautiful women. In Lebanon, punching the left palm with a closed right fist is a sign of flirtation. Unlike other societies which have strict taboos against affectionate male physical contact, in Arab and many Mediterranean countries it is common to see men walk hand in hand as a gesture of friendship. And all Arabs stand close together and frequently touch each other during conversation. However, the gesturing of the Arab is always done with the right hand, as opposed to the "unclean" left.

SIGN LANGUAGE OF THE DEAF

Paul Tabori, in his *Book of the Hand,* tells of a slander case in Wales where both the plaintiff and the defendant were deaf and dumb. And the slander was actually committed (the defendant had to pay substantial damages) in their sign language.

FINGERPRINTS

Because we know that fingerprints are as individual as snow-flakes, the fingerprint is evidence that this is the only shot you get at being you.

HANDS IN ART

Painting and sculpting hands present a difficult challenge to the artist, and because poor hand representation can mar an otherwise fine work of art, painters and sculptors meticulously study the workings of the hand. Among the many famous hands in art are those of the sculptures of Rodin and Da Vinci's painting of Mona Lisa, whose hands are written about almost as much as her smile.

Many famous pieces of sculpture survive even though the original hands created by the artist have broken off, such as those of the Venus de Milo. The hands of a statue are fragile, and vulnerable to destruction.

HANDS AND THE PERFORMING ARTS

Some actors avoid having their hands show in film closeups. I can't remember ever seeing Grace Kelly's hands featured, except in white gloves, which became a trademark of her elegant image. (It was rumored that she was a nail biter). But Rita Hayworth's hands were magnificent and always evident. Ironically, having elegant hands actually "handicapped" actress Sylvia Sydney when being cast for a role as a lower-class woman on a TV film. Theatrical agent Michael Hartig told me that the director rejected Sydney for the role of a factory seamstress because he felt that her perfect hands and nails would render the character unbelievable. Sydney cut her long nails, returned "unpolished" and got the job. Furthermore, she so perfected the character, down to the fingertips, that much of the show consisted of tight closeups of her hands.

•

French pantomimist Marcel Marceau moves his hands to portray movement and emotion as a painter uses a brush to make his artistic statement. Masters of sleight of hand, like Houdini and card wizard John Scarne, develop such dexterity that their hands move faster than the eye can follow.

•

The late film director Alfred Hitchcock was a master at using hand closeups for exposition of plot and character. In *Dial M for Murder*, we watch every step of the crime, but only through the murderer's hands. Who actually dunnit doesn't become evident until the last reel.

Actress Jessie Royce Landis, playing Grace Kelly's wealthy mother in Hitchcock's *To Catch a Thief*, snuffs out her cigarette in a runny egg yolk, thereby betraying her coarse upbringing.

•

Robert Dailey, producer of Clint Eastwood's films (and coincidentally collector of rare hand manuscripts) told me that the fast draw, so popular in movie and TV Westerns, is actually a gimmick invented for movies, and never appeared in authentic Wild West lore. The only shooting done by cowboys and Indians was in the back or during an ambush.

•

Some directors don't like to use "insert shots." Arthur Hiller, director of *Love Story*, *The Out-of-Towners*, and *The In-Laws*, told me how he solved the problem when he directed *Love Story*, in which the character of Jennifer, played by Ali McGraw, was a concert pianist. Since McGraw didn't play the piano, he designed this one piano scene so that she would be required to actually play the piano for only seventeen seconds. However, it was necessary for the producers to send her to a piano teacher, and it took her three weeks of concentrated study to acquire enough skill to perform the seventeen-second shot.

•

Because stage acting requires exaggerated or gross movements which are often inappropriate for the screen closeup, stage actors occasionally encounter difficulty bringing their gestures "down" for movies and TV. Conversely, screen actors often can't be "big" enough for the stage.

Tony Curtis in an interview described the challenge to the screen actor of handling a coffeecup so that his nose isn't obscured for the camera, placing it down on the exact marks to insure a perfectly framed shot, all the while remembering his lines, as well as keeping his "intention" and emotional condition for a scene.

HANDS IN DANCE

Temple dancers of the Orient, hypnotic Hawaiian dancers and classical ballerinas are all trained to use their hands in their art. The primary use of the hands in most dance forms is to complete the line of the dancer's body. Exotic gestures of Oriental temple dancers often feature the hands held in profile vertically over the head, providing a frame for the head as it is extended from side to side by extreme extensions of the neck.

George Balanchine is reputed to be a taskmaster regarding the position of every finger of a dancer's hand. A famous ballerina noted that she takes the trouble to specifically position her pinky "for Mr. B." The limp, graceful ballet hand contrasts dramatically with the forceful flexing of the hand in modern dance.

Janet Eilber, star of the Martha Graham troupe, told me that whether she is making the sign of the cross for "Joan of Arc" or the clawed hand of "Cassandra," her goal is to have the hand gesture emanate from the center of the body, falling into a position that best expresses the drama, with the energy coming out of the heel of the hand.

Hula dancing, which is known as much for sinuously swaying hips as for its hypnotic hand gestures, was originally performed in a kneeling position, utilizing only hands and facial expressions. According to the writings of Tanao Sands, hula (or hula-hula, as it was called for emphasis) is "the act of personifying the meaning of a word."

Since the ancient Polynesians had no written form of communication, the hand gesture assumed great importance in their culture. Along with chanting, hula was developed as a means of chronicling and extolling. Although hula later developed into a theatrical dance form, it was this original high intention that accounted for the fact that early hula dancers were temple novitiates. They were separated from the community and allowed to engage in special activities in order to empower their hands. In addition to working the hands under water and performing exercises that simulated water pressure, hula dancers were constantly tested on other forms of control of their hands. In order to keep their hands supple, they did the honey exercise described on pages 184-185.

Thumbs and Lovers

The man facing me picked up his drink. When I looked at his thumb I knew he could kill me. I later discovered that in fact he was divorced by his wife on the grounds of severe physical abuse. Little Jack Horner of the nursery rhyme knew what he was doing when he used his thumb to get the plum he wanted. The thumb is a good indication of a person's basic energy, and its size, shape, and how it's held can speak volumes. Forceful use of the thumbs in gestures intensifies the speaker's point, as in pointing the thumb to the self when indicating "I." Use of the thumb pointing away from the self not only indicates direction, but also provides added information. It is the silent equivalent of "Beat it, chum." When a person is trying to shape

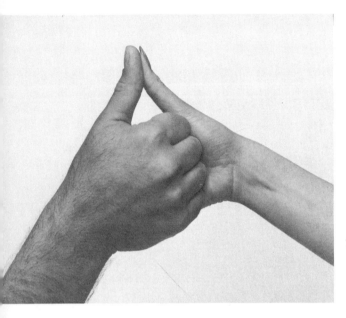

Thumb wrestling

a thought he will often hold the thumb and forefinger close to each other, but not actually touching, in an effort to "feel for" or confine the thought that he is attempting to verbalize. This gesture is performed with the thumb toward the speaker, and the whole hand moving slightly in the direction of the listener, giving an almost "trumpet" effect to the words. Singers some-times use this gesture to indicate that they are refining and perfecting a musical sound. If, however, that same gesture is done with the thumb held in the direction of the listener, lightly shaking up and down, it is telling you that, even if the speaker is asking for something, he is still in control. This is a gesture often used by Italians to emphasize a point. They are telling you that their thumb is "on top of things."

How a person holds his thumb indicates not only how much energy he has but also how he will use it. Palmists consider the thumb to represent the will. Babies usually hide their thumbs with their fingers, but if they throw a temper tantrum, the thumb comes out, showing self-assertion. It has been observed that just before an epileptic seizure, the victim pulls his thumb in, covering it with the fingers. A person whose hands are fisted with the thumb on top of the fingers is hostile and literally ready to punch. Notice the position of the thumbs of people you are negotiating with. If your opponent's thumbs are covered by his fingers, he is licked before he starts. For confidence, you, on the other hand, can keep your courage up by keeping your thumbs out. So if you are asking for something, keep on top of things by making sure your thumbs are not covered by your fingers.

A person who generally holds his thumbs away from his hands is generous and open with his thoughts, feelings and gifts. The person who is more guarded holds his thumb close to his fingers. And I am always fascinated to see how a man moves his thumb. Whether it moves decisively with the hand or just idles around nervously tells me much about his feelings about himself and the world. I once knew a man who would silently rehearse or sometimes relive entire arguments with other people by moving his thumbs.

A thumb that bends back easily at the joint is usually a sign of a person who rolls with the punches. He or she can be versatile, brilliant and extremely generous—also overly extravagant, restless and have difficulty finishing anything. If nothing else, these people are great starters. The stiff thumb is found on the hand of the practical, economical, cautious and steady person. These people usually don't make the splash of those with supple thumbs, but are more realistic and more likely to be satisfied with a quiet life, or at least to attempt to maintain a low profile concerning their activities.

A large thumb indicates strength of character, and its owner is usually capable and forceful. The small-thumbed person is guided by sentiment and romance. The person who has a small, stiff thumb is a quibbler.

A thumb which is fairly broad at the nail but nicely waisted at the joint is a sign that the person is strong, healthy and tactful. If, however, the thumb is extremely waisted, be on guard against someone who is tactful to the point of lying. If the thumb has the same thickness all the way up (sometimes resembling a cocktail frankfurter) the person can be a stubborn, blunt, coarse and brutal lover. He just doesn't stop to reason. A pinched look to the fingertip is often a sign of nervousness. A thumb with a short first joint with a puffed tip that looks like a knob usually indicates a violent temper. Palmists sometimes refer to this type as a "murderer's thumb." While this is certainly not concrete evidence of criminality, I am always on the lookout when I see this "clubbed" thumb on a hand that has short fingers (signifying quick action), coarse texture (insensitivity), very thick third phalages (sensuality) and deep red lines in the hand (swift flow of energy). If crossed, a person with such a thumb is capable of beating your brains out.

•

Anthropologists correlate the development of the thumb with the evolution of the human cerebral cortex (the reason for the human's superior cognitive functioning). The hands of gorillas and chimpanzees, which bear considerable resemblance to the human hand, have thumbs that are small, set low and at a considerable distance from the rest of the fingers. The human ability to execute thumb opposition (i.e., placing the thumb pad to the pad of any other finger, especially the little finger) is the most complex and refined in the entire body. We probably have right or left "thumbedness" as well as handedness.

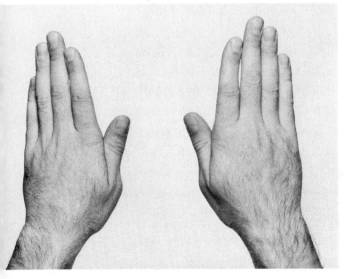

Guarded thumbs

Simple Handreading

O N EXAMINING anyone's hands, including your own, bear in mind that a combination of traits gives accurate character assessment, and the appearance of any quality in the hand must be verified in at least two tests to have any validity. And remember, any feature of the hands can be changed or modified to a striking degree.

THE RIGHT AND THE LEFT HAND

Note that palmists consider the left hand (in a right-handed person) to represent the unconscious life as well as the person's potential. The right hand represents what is actual, how an individual has handled his problems, or how easy or difficult it has been for him to follow his original "life path."

TEXTURE

Texture is determined by feeling the skin on the back of the hand. It is the key to the natural refinement of the person. The difference in the texture of the two hands can reveal much about a person's social mobility. If the left is rough while the right is smoother, the person has attained some refinement. Very fine texture tells that the person just can't say "So what!" These people are oversensitive to what others do and say about them, no matter how tough their demeanor. Very fine texture can be found on the hands of those who do the roughest tasks, and conversely, rough texture can be found on young and (seemingly) refined boarding school students.

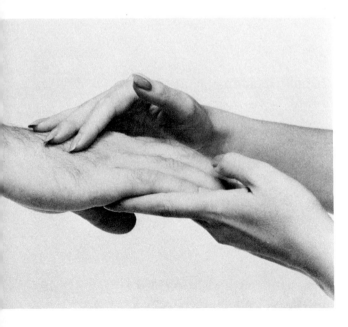

Feeling for skin texture

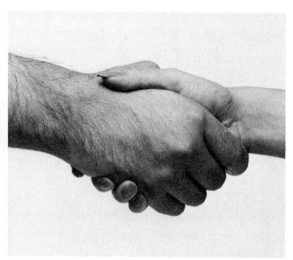

Consistency

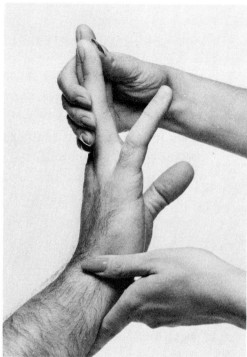

Test for flexibility

CONSISTENCY

The degree of elasticity of the muscles of the hand indicates the flexibility or rigidity of the personality. If, as you shake the hand, the hand grips and releases as you release, the person is usually intelligent, trustworthy and full of energy. The person with hard consistency has tremendous physical energy but is not at all cerebral. The person with weak consistency has low energy and is hard to stir to activity. This is why we are often turned off by the "dead fish" handshake.

FLEXIBILITY

If the fingers are stiff, so is the person. An argument with him is an exercise in futility. He lives in the past, isn't receptive to new ideas, tends to hoard old possessions, and is narrow in his outlook. The owner of the flexible hand is versatile and mentally adaptable. But if the fingers are very flexible, the person is often weak-willed and overly susceptible to other's ideas. What we look for are medium qualities in these tests. Also, you can begin to see that if a person has hard consistency and lack of flexibility in his hands, he is more rigid than the person with hard consistency and flexible fingers.

COLOR

The color of the palm is an indication of the temperament and health of the person, and is directly related to the bloodstream. Most palms are a shade of pink. The white-palmed person may be cold and distant; he lacks sensuality, is dreamy and mystical and makes few friends. Red palms signify intensity of physical expression. These people are ardent. Yellow color signifies a cynical pessimist who can be sarcastic and moody. He always crosses bridges before he gets there and can be very uncooperative. Blue color is usually seen after illness or surgery.

NAILS

Nails give us an insight into the robustness and sensitivity of the person. They are like windows. Look for smooth, pliable nails without bumps, fluting or scaling. Any variation shows us something is out of balance.

Any mark, be it a white dot or a knife mark, shows that a serious physical or emotional upheaval has occurred. The timing of the event is told by the location of the mark. It takes six months for a nail to grow out, so if the mark occurs in the middle of the nail, the event took place three months ago.

The shape of the nail gives us more information. A narrow nail, compared to the width of the whole fleshy part of the finger, shows a lack of robustness. Nervous energy keeps these people going. The broad nail is usually a sign of muscular strength and energy. The deep or long nail (from cuticle to tip) belongs to the frank person. If the nail is deep as well as broad, the person is open and easy to get along with. Medium-short nails often tell of a quizzical nature. However, very short nails, especially if bitten, reveal a very critical personality. The criticism is often turned towards the self, and, if the cuticle is also ragged, he is literally "running himself ragged."

FINGERTIPS

The general rule is the more pointed the tip the more idealistic the person; the broader the tip, the more practical. The spatulate tip, the broadest, wants action, is on the go and is extremely enthusiastic. Conic tips suggest artistic, impulsive people who rely more on intuition than on reasoning.

Noted palmist Frank Andrews told me that most babies have spatulate fingertips, showing their freedom and openness. During the school years, the tips tend to change and become squared as the children are expected to accept a certain amount of dogma by rote. As they mature, however, it is not uncommon for the tips to become more conic or rounded as the individual creativity develops and is allowed to express itself. If the person becomes extremely religious his fingertips may become pointed, showing the least resistance to divine inspiration.

Andrews illustrated the distinctions between the varying fingertips by describing the sort of artwork that might be done by each type. The artist with spatulate fingertips would paint a horse running through a field. The feeling would be expansive, and the canvas probably large. The artist with square tips would paint the horse standing still and would include lots of detail in his picture. The artist with conic tips would create a painting of a very beautiful horse, using lots of color to illustrate its magnificence. However, the artist with pointed fingertips would see his horse with wings and would possibly depict him as a flying horse. Picasso had spatulate and squared fingertips, and was, of course, one of the pioneers of the cubist style of painting.

SMOOTH AND KNOTTED JOINTS

All of us have two joints on each finger and one on the thumb. People with pronounced joints or knots are neat, lead orderly lives, and are the doubting Thomases of the world. The more pronounced the knot, the more philosophical, slow-acting and less likely to be led they are. Overmeticulousness is thought by some to cause arthritis. If you have smooth fingers, you may develop knots later if your personality becomes overly judgmental.

LONG AND SHORT FINGERS

People with long fingers go into the smallest details. They don't accept change easily and are offended at the drop of a hat. The short-fingered person despises detail. He thinks big, quickly, and considers the whole picture. Don't give him details; give him results. He is intuitive and gets to the point. Often he is a fast talker and may be impulsive and hotheaded.

WORLDS

The hand as a whole is divided into three worlds: the mental, the practical, and the material or sensual. Because it is rare to find a balanced hand, one or two worlds usually predominate. If the fingers are very long, the mental world predominates. A large middle section (the area from where the thumb is attached

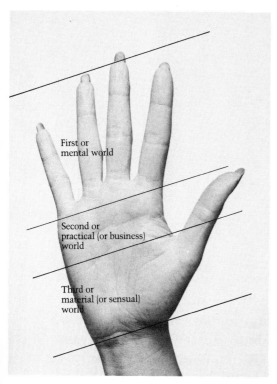

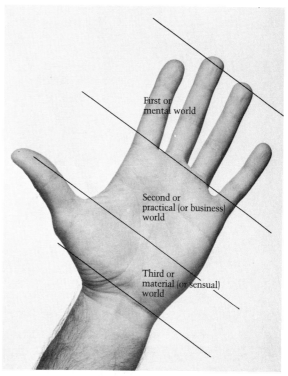

Hand with large first and third worlds   Hand with large second world

to its webbing up to the base of the fingers) belongs to the person who is interested in practical matters; he is your businessman. If the third world (from the thumb to the wrist, that is, the heel of the hand) is large, the person wants results and is quite capable of asking for what he wants. He is also usually a physically oriented person. Professional people often have prominent first and third worlds. And the wise ones leave the business side of their work to others. A person with little third world is not asking enough from life, both materially and emotionally.

THE LINES

The lines of the hand show the details of one's life. When events have strongly impressed themselves upon the brain, lines ap-

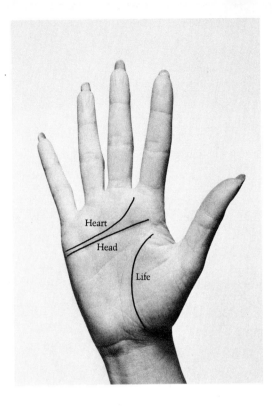

The three major lines

pear. However, if someone makes a dire prediction about you because of a line in your hand, run, do not walk to the nearest exit. Lines can change in as little as three weeks, when you change your point of view, and thus your destiny.

In general, the deeper and clearer the lines in your hand, the clearer your path will be. And please note that the length of the life line does not necessarily determine how long you will live! The curve of it, however, can tell a lot about a person's love life. A very curved life line, sweeping into the palm, outlining a large cushion or heel of the hand attached to the thumb, usually belongs to a lustful, healthy, good-natured, warm person. A life line that cleaves close to the thumb, with a fairly flat heel, can be the sign of a person who is more mental than physical, is shy, and tends to have relationships that are more platonic than sexual.

THE MOUNDS

The prominence or absence of mounds tells us much about the character, preferences and dilemmas of the person. For example, a large or prominent mound under the finger of Jupiter (the pointer finger) suggests a leader, one who uses his voice effectively to influence people, who can be an overprotective parent, is predisposed to drinking problems, and should only marry a person he is proud of. Now if the subject also has a prominent mound of Venus (the cushiony portion attached to the thumb) he can be very attracted to a lover because of lust. Thus a conflict is present. He may be crazy about a woman because of their physical relationship, but if he isn't proud of her, a marriage between them will never work.

The interesting part of this study really begins when the different worlds and tests are placed together. Not only does each finger represent different character qualities, but also the phalanx of each finger. Now, consider that the lines in your hands can actually change within three weeks. Mounds and phalanxes can change within months—I can personally bear witness to that.

THE SIMIAN LINE

When the heart and head lines are fused, as on a monkey's palm, the existing line is called the "simian" line. Although this is often evidence of mongoloidism in infants, palmists believe that it can be a sign of genius as well. It is also thought to indicate intensity and is not uncommon on the hands of people who agonize and have overly possessive attitudes.

THE PALM LINES AS DIAGNOSTIC TOOL

At the Children's Medical Research Foundation in Sydney, Australia, Dr. Margaret A. Menser and S. G. Purvis-Smith identified what they call the "Sydney line," an extended head line that becomes a simianlike crease, slanting across the palm, but leaving a separate heart line. The investigators found that 36 percent of the children studied suffering from leukemia had either the simian or Sydney lines in one or both palms (as against 13 percent of normal children).

A VISIT TO THREE PALMISTS

Florens Meschter was the protégé of the late William Benham, author of the most widely used textbook on palmistry, *The Laws of Scientific Hand Reading*. The first thing she will tell you is that there is nothing in your hands that you can't change. Lines can change in three weeks, and even the mounds under the fingers, which reveal character traits, can change or disappear entirely if there is a corresponding change in the personality. The second declaration Mrs. Meschter makes is that she is no fortune teller. She feels that the value of her work is in character analysis and vocational guidance, as opposed to foretelling future events. Claiming to have no psychic ability, she reads the hand as a doctor would examine an X-ray. She begins with simple flexibility and texture tests, proceeds to meticulously measure each phalanx of all the fingers, then takes prints of the various areas of each palm. Only after careful analysis of the findings, which are recorded on your chart, will she begin to give you any information about yourself. Her intention is to encourage the subject to use the talents he has and become aggressive in developing those that are lacking or underdeveloped, as graphically noted in the hand.

•

Mr. Singh came from India to New York in 1970. Since childhood he had been aware that he was different from others in how he perceived events. He vowed that he wouldn't charge for his perceptions until he read ten thousand hands, as payment to the universe for his gift. He has now read the palms of count-less famous entertainers and politicians as well as thousands of "civilians." Singh also considers himself a healer, and uses the vibrations he receives from the person to aid communication with the subject's "true spirit." He will tell you of past lives your soul has experienced (often as animals or vegetation, as well as human forms), and considers the intimates in your pres-ent life to be the reincarnation of unfinished karmic relation-ships in your past lives.

●

Frank Andrews, who has been referred to as the "Rolls-Royce of Readers," is the darling of many famous celebrities. Andrews is so well known in certain circles that his presence at a party has sent otherwise friendly people to the opposite side of the room in order to sit on their hands, lest they reveal too much of themselves to his discerning eye.

Andrews, who is a psychic as well, also uses Tarot cards during a "reading." He told me that while the Tarot tells him the "now" or the "probably," the hands reveal the overall pic-ture, or "climate" of the person.

Although some clients are men, it is mostly women who seek out his services. Though more and more women come to him for career advice, the most common dilemmas are still "af-fairs of the heart." Andrews views his hardest task as "to be free of judgment regarding each person's case." His goal is to "act like a camera and just see the picture without giving an opinion of the picture."

He admitted that the only case he ever read incorrectly was that of a psychotic, a man whom he saw "professionally" over a three-year period. Andrews explained that this extraordinary happenstance could occur only because the subject actually be-lieved his lies, and therefore his hands never revealed the phon-iness of his true character.

The Laying on of Hands

HEALING THROUGH TOUCH—the laying on of hands—is a spiritual or psychic healing method that was said in the Bible to have been performed by Jesus. While mainly a phenomenon known to Protestant sects, it is currently practiced by some Hasidic groups, and in the Charismatic Catholic movement, which is growing in constituency. Most spiritual healers claim to be a channel through which God or Jesus, the Christ consciousness, or a "higher" or "universal" consciousness passes energy for healing.

The healer places his hand on the person afflicted, claiming to plug into a universal energy, as one plugs an electric light into a socket. The universal energy is then transferred to the ailing one in order to assist him to cut the connection to the illness.

It has been said of me that when I perform a healing procedure on another person, the energies that emanate from my hands can actually be felt.

WHO CAN HEAL?

There are two schools of thought. One is that it is a natural rather than a developed skill. The other is that all of us have the potential to be healers, just as all of us can sing, but some do it better than others (and some respond better to some amount of training and focus). I tend to subscribe to the latter theory. Most mothers have had the experience of touching a child and somehow knowing that he is sick, even if his body is cool to the touch. The importance of "hugging" is now becoming a respectable part of some forms of personality therapy, as a result of studies of the aberrated psyches and impaired physical development of babies raised in orphanages who have been deprived of loving touch. The strong emotional connection or "love link" to a child or lover empowers our touch, and such touching enables us all to perform major or minor miracles.

FAMOUS HEALERS' HANDS

Healer Kathryn Kulman claimed to have ordinary hands which "happened to do God's work," whereas others claim to have hands possessing special powers. Conversely, Marjoe Gortner claims his "talent," when he was a child evangelist, was a hoax encouraged by the religious equivalent of a stage mother (although many claim to have been cured by his hands).

KIRLIAN PHOTOGRAPHY

Through the development of Kirlian photography, sometimes referred to as radiation field photography, energies that emanate from the fingertips have been recorded. Kirlian photographs of Krivorotov taken in the Soviet Union and of Ethel de Louch taken here (by Professor E. Douglas Dean of Newark College of Engineering) show extraordinary bursts of energy during the act of healing.

DOCTORS AS HEALERS

The current medical opinion supports the position that a doctor provides the body with procedures to enable it to heal itself. In addition to their superior sense of touch, rendering them superior diagnosticians, most effective doctors are actually "healers." Their vision of the patient remains at the highest potential, and can effect the fastest and most expedient recovery for the patient.

MASSAGE

When a mother rubs a child's bruise, she shows an instinctive knowledge of healing. Massage releases physical and emotional toxins, increases circulation, reduces swelling, blood pressure and pain, and releases energy. Healing through massage, an aspect of ancient health science, dates back to Hippocrates (400 B.C.). Oriental massage is often done by applying pressure to the face and other parts of the body with the thumbs. Zone therapy (or reflexology) in its various forms assumes that various points of the face, feet and hands correspond to the internal organs, and therefore applying pressure to these points results in reduction of toxicity from those organs.

The Kama Sutra, the ancient Indian manual of sex procedures, describes different kinds of pinches, scratches and rubbing gestures used to release sexual energies from different terminals of the body.

Lomi lomi, a Hawaiian method of massage derived from ancient Polynesia, is rather like kneading dough, differing from the stroking, rubbing or pressing massage techniques of Sweden and other cultures. The kneading action of lomi lomi relaxes and heals by drawing the energies through the body from the extremities to the sexual center. Diners in a restaurant on a Polynesian island will often find an item called "lomi lomi salmon" on the menu. It literally means "massaged" or "broken-up" salmon.

TOUCH

The sense of touch enables us to "hear" and "see" with our hands. The nerve apparatus of touch lies immediately under the skin's surface. The tips of the tactile nerves are sandwiched in between a dozen small cells, which are covered by a membrane. When pressure is applied at the fingertips, the ends of the "wires" touch and a nerve current passes along to the brain. The fingertips have more of these concentrated nerve cables, and are more closely spaced, than in any other part of the body except the tongue. (Palmists note that very sensitive people have "sensitive pads" on one or more fingertips.) And so communication by touch is dependent on pressure and vibration, which is how Helen Keller learned to speak and "hear."

The development of the tactile sense is dependent on experience and talent. Doctors' fingers are often so educated that they can be as sensitive as a stethoscope in detecting areas of congestion in a patient's body. In a similar way, masseuses and masseurs, chiropractors and other professionals who manipulate the body to promote health have a highly developed sense of touch. Card sharks and burglars often file down the surface of

STOCKINGS

the skin to increase the sensitivity of their fingertips.

Superstar hair stylist Kenneth Battelle, who rose to fame "when a client of mine went to the White House" told me: "I cut hair as much by touch as by eye, which is why I can't teach hair cutting."

BRAILLE

The Braille alphabet starts with A and ends with Z, followed by the comma, period and only then the letter W. This is because Louis Braille was French, and the French language has no W. In addition to the alphabet, there is a Braille "shorthand" for many words, as well as musical notations.

Pianist George Shearing, blind since birth, has actually turned a handicap into an asset. The increased sensitivity of his hearing and touch have undoubtedly added to his artistry.

Keeping an extensive tape catalogue and carefully indexed card file (all of which, including equipment switches, are labeled in Braille), Shearing can locate all the material and operate all the elaborate sound equipment in his studio without assistance. When I commented on the meticulous order of everything in the studio, he replied, "A blind man has to be neat."

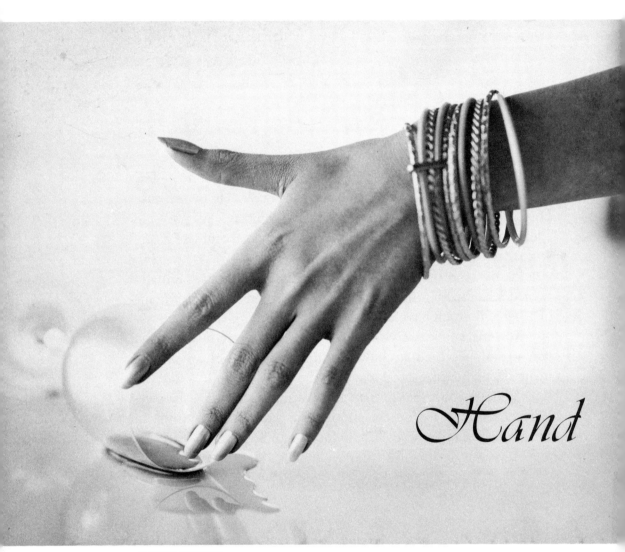

Hand

STANLEY JOHNSON

Health and Beauty

Professional Repair
for Broken and Split Nails

COUNTLESS PEOPLE ask me what I do when I break a nail. I usually say, "Cry a lot!" Actually, because I cook and sew and do most of the activities that people who don't earn their living from "manual labor" do, I am usually walking around with a few mended nails (and even occasionally a repair of a complete break-off). Over the years I have discovered some terrific mending techniques that are waterproof, and more importantly, embarrassment-proof. And if you use the mending techniques as soon as you notice a weakening at the side of the nail, or a slight tear, complete replacement of a broken nail will rarely be necessary.

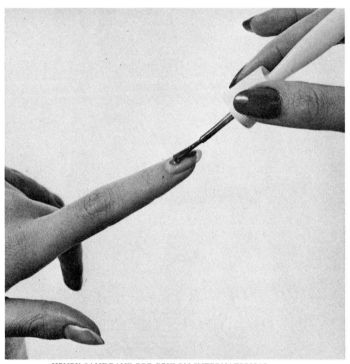

HENRY SANDBANK FOR REVLON INTERNATIONAL

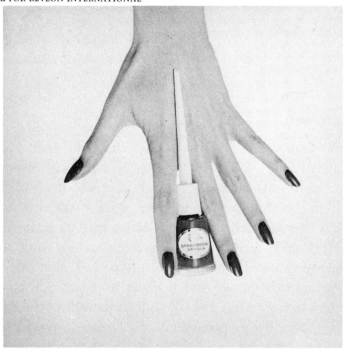

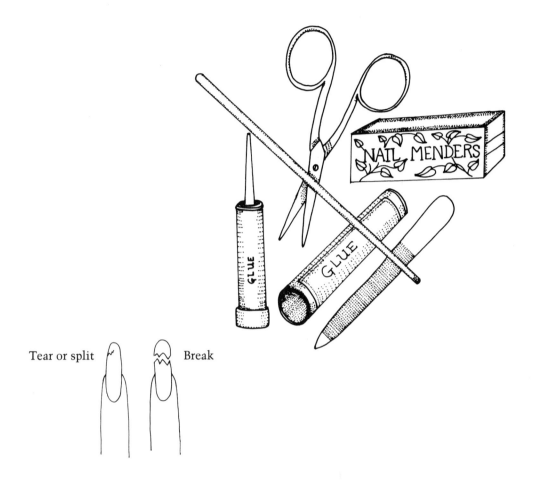

Tear or split   Break

TO REPAIR SPLITS

Crazy Glue or Five-Second Glue

These glues can be applied to a split in your nail, or used to reaffix a broken-off one (more below). Use sparingly, as this glue bonds instantly and drips will harden into bumps on your nail (or skin for that matter, if you are really careless). Also, this strong chemical can weaken the surface of the nail plate, so apply judiciously, avoiding any unnecessary spill onto the nail surface.

To apply, have another person gently lift the broken part of

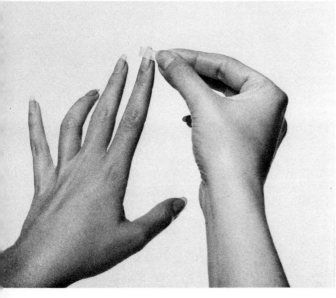

1. Trim paper so it fits over break

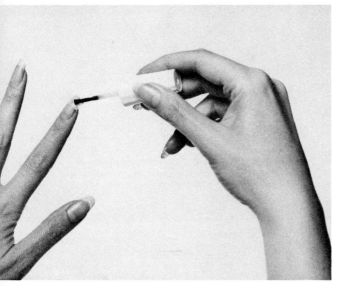

2. Use loaded nail-mender brush to apply paper to the nail

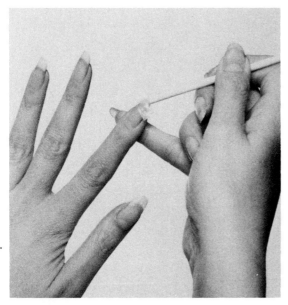

3. Wrap paper under nail

the nail with an orange stick and apply the glue sparingly to both *inside* edges of the nail. Press the two pieces together.

Special Mender Procedure

For most splits and breaks I strongly recommend the following method, perfected for me by Jean Rayner, a very successful hand model from England.

You can begin with Crazy Glue or not, depending on how bad the split or break is and how much heavy duty your hands are required to do. I used this method for years before the invention of Crazy Glue, but the glue does add strength to your "patch." With or without Crazy Glue, it is the best, safest and most aesthetically appealing method I know to avoid what used to be disaster for me.

1. Use one of the "nail-mender kits" such as Revlon or Max Factor.

2. Always start with clean, oil-free and lotion-free nails.

3. Cut a strip of nail-mender paper large enough so that it will cover your break (1) and wrap under the tip of your nail. Apply a coat of the liquid mender to the bare nail. Using the brush applicator provided, saturate the mender paper with the liquid. Then apply the saturated paper to the break (2). Wrap it as smoothly as you can with an orange stick (3). Tuck the extra paper under the nail to give it added strength. *Note:* If the break is just a small one, I will tuck less paper under the nail because the extra support isn't necessary, and the paper often gets "mushy" after a few days and has to be replaced.

4. As the surface dries, you may notice a few more bumps. Dip the tip of the index finger of your opposite hand in remover, and then smooth the surface of the wrapped nail.

5. Let dry a few minutes and reapply a coat of nail-mender liquid. Let dry a few minutes again and repeat the finger-smoothing process. Repeat the nail mender liquid application and finger smoothing process one more time. This will give your nail a smooth, hard surface. If the break is extreme, you may

want to repeat all of this with an additional piece of mending paper that you place in the opposite direction of the first (i.e., horizontally).

6. If possible, let the nail dry overnight before applying nail enamel.

Cotton Patches

A small piece of cotton rolled at the sides and tucked under the nail gives even greater strength than nail-mender paper but is a little more difficult to apply yourself. Some manicurists recommend fine handkerchief linen for this process. Famous manicurist Nina Ricco uses coffee-filter paper instead because she finds it thinner. The above procedure can be used with any of these.

Emergency Repair for Completely Broken Off Nail

If you split a nail and don't have mender or paper, you can saturate a small piece of facial tissue with base coat or clear polish. Apply to your nail, as above. It should hold you till you can use one of the stronger aids.

TO REPAIR NAIL BREAKS

What if your nail breaks off completely? Dry your tears immediately so you can look for the lost tip!

1. You can glue it back on with Crazy Glue. If the tip has dried out, soak it in some warm water till it's pliable.

2. If you don't have your own tip, you can buy a product like Eve'n Tips. These are the same tips that many salons use for extensions, or porcelains. File the tip to the desired length (these are sold outrageously long). Apply with Crazy Glue, using the method described above.

3. Do not stop at this point. The glue is too strong to give

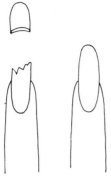

Eve'n Tip

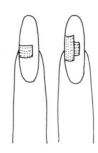

Fibrous mending paper

your new nail tip and the supporting part of your nail plate the proper balance. A pull on that nail tip can result in a break way below the quick.

4. Get out your trusty nail-mender kit and use the procedure for mending described above. However, instead of one horizontal paper in wrapping, also run two vertical strips of mending paper at both sides of the nail to provide extra strength.

Special Emergency Repair to Get You Through the Night

My manicurist, Hae Young, helped me devise this special technique. If your nail is badly split or completely broken off, glue back the nail with Crazy Glue or Five-Second Glue. Hold together for a few seconds until the bonding is secure. Then take a piece of plastic tape or Scotch brand Magic Mending Tape cut to the shape needed to strip across the break, and apply with further application of Crazy Glue.

Use the fine side of an emery board or some very fine sandpaper to gently smooth down the edges of the plastic tape so that the edges won't be noticeable when covered by polish.

Alternative: Cut a strip of mending tape to cover the break and apply. Then take Crazy Glue and apply sparingly along the edges of the tape. Smooth as above.

ACRYLIC MENDER KITS

These kits are sold to repair split or broken nails. I have found the chemicals in most of these kits (an acrylic powder and a solvent) too strong to recommend. The "paste" they are mixed into can weaken the nail, increasing the probability of breakage as the nail grows out. The chemicals can also cause allergic reactions and fungus infections, so use them only if you are a nail biter—acrylics are probably less injurious to your nail bed than biting your nails.

FALSE NAILS

The advantage of false nails is that they are cheap and can be applied faster than any other remedy for the broken nail. The arguments against their use are that the glue provided must be applied to the entire nail surface (and so can rob the nail plate of natural oils and weaken the nail), and that false nails fall off more readily than nails repaired in other ways.

Soften false nails in warm water before you use them to facilitate bending them into the shape. The glue that usually comes with these kits isn't that strong (which is for your protection) so don't keep them on too long. The glue can give, and nothing looks tackier than an otherwise beautifully turned-out woman lifting a long-stemmed goblet with a hand sporting only four long red nails. It's usually the pointer that goes first, too.

I can't seem to do business with false nails, though some of my competitors can. The very same blessing of long, narrowly shaped nails makes commercial false nails look like toenails on my hand. I can, however, usually get away with them on all but my thumb and pointer fingers, as these are likely to be focused too close for comfort by the camera. When I do use false nails, I apply them with double-faced tape, so that they can be easily removed after the shoot.

TO GET FRAGILE NAILS TO GROW

The following methods should help you grow long nails if you have never been able to grow them before.

The Nail Wrap or "Juliette"

This is the only procedure I can recommend without reservation that covers and protects fragile nails. This method was developed by Juliette Marglen, was popularized in Los Angeles, and is now flourishing in salons all over the country. With practice, you can master this process on your own nails to give them extra support.

Use one of the nail-mender kits that contain mending liquid and papers. Cut all the papers you will need before beginning application, and make sure there are no traces of oil or lotion on your nails. The "cover" should be wedge-shaped and fit over your nail, extending about ⅛ inch over the edge all around the

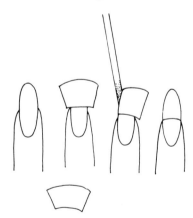

1. Cut wedge
2. Place on nail tip
3. Wrap under sides with orange stick

tip. A special trick taught me by my manicurist, Hae Young, is to prick the surface of the mending tissue with a straight pin in several places to allow the air to escape and reduce the possibility of bubbling. Saturate the paper in the liquid and then brush the nail surface with the same liquid. Tuck the end under the nail and smooth with an orange stick. Dip the stick into remover and try to remove all wrinkles and lumps. Let dry and

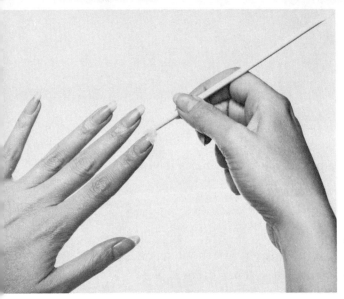

The nail wrap helps fragile nails grow

apply base coat, then clear or colored enamel. You can also add a sealer, which is colorless, and coat the underside of the nail.

Acrylic Sculptures

The sculptured nail was invented in the Hollywood movie studio to make a star's less-than-perfect hands more glamorous. It is relatively recently that they have been available to all, in salons or home kits. Patti Nail appeared on the market in the late fifties, but was removed because some of its ingredients were found to be harmful. However the name "Patti Nail" has become synonymous with the acrylic sculptures that are being done today. There are do-it-yourself kits available, but this requires such dexterity that most women who wear acrylic nails have them done at a salon specializing in nail work. First the nail surface is roughed up with sandpaper or an emery board so that the acrylic paste will grip. The acrylic is actually a powder and a solvent which is applied wet over your own nail, and further extended over horseshoe-shaped silver paper forms. When dry, the silver papers are removed and the hardened surface is smoothed with an emergy board and fine sandpaper. The more conscientious salons apply the acrylic to the upper portion of the nail only, leaving the lower part free to "breathe." Porcelains or "extensions," as they are sometimes called, employ similar acrylic paste. Here a plastic tip is glued onto the edge of your nail with Crazy Glue, and the acrylic is then layered over the nail and tip.

These processes can take from one and a half to three hours. New York manicurist Moi has admitted to spending six and a half hours perfecting nails on perfectionist Faye Dunaway for one of her film roles. These nails can set you back $45 to $100, depending on where you have them done and precisely which method is used. And once on, these require fill ins to be done every two weeks or so. These cost about $3 to $5 per nail. Complete removal is about $20.00.

Should you take the plunge and give yourself instant nail glamour at all costs? Aside from the expense, doctors caution of the possible dangers. Roughing up the nail in the preparation stage removes a layer or layers of nail and strips the surface of moisture. The paste itself can cause fungus infections and allergic reactions. Representatives from Revlon Research Labs told me they were horrified to learn that some nail emporiums were mixing up acrylic formulas which contained Revlon enamel solvent, a product developed for use in thinning enamels, but never tested for use in combination with these other chemicals.

Still, many women swear by acrylics, never encounter a problem, even after years of use, and love the glamour and convenience of their new seemingly strong nails. And, while it is true that doctors only get to see people with problems, even those salons who tout the application of acrylics usually recommend that they be removed twice a year to give your nails a rest. I found removal of these to be difficult and at times painful, and the nail underneath weaker and dryer than before. It also takes six months to a year to grow out the weakened part. That is if you are lucky and have had no damage to the nail bed. It's too big a risk for my money, but if you have very weak nails to begin with, you may want to chance it.

Fads, Fashions and
Famous Manicurists

WHEN LIZA MINNELLI painted her nails emerald green for her role as the "divinely decadent" Sally Bowles in *Cabaret,* nail enamel companies had a good, if unexpected, rise in sales of green polish for several months. The same thing happened when Cher painted her fabulously long, squared-off nails green for a segment of her TV show. What is considered outrageous at one time may be quite acceptable at another. Red nails, once denounced as "unnatural," were popularized in the forties by movie stars, whose blood-red nails often photographed black before the widespread use of technicolor. (Hand modeling almost always calls for pale-pink colors so that those who are watching black-and-white TV will not perceive the nails as overly dark, thereby calling unwanted attention to the tone of the polish.)

During the sixties, the desire of the flower children to "let it all hang out" resulted in the trend toward flesh tones and translucent polishes. The current popularity of red nails is actually a throwback to the forties, along with other nostalgic fashion trends. Leaving the "moon" exposed at the base of the nails is another popular revival. Enamel shades ranging from brown-toned to oxblood are in. But then Egyptian women painted not only their nails, but also their palms red with henna!

Pop art inspired a new look for nails. Tina Sinatra sported black, blue, purple and yellow checks painted on her nails. Linda Lovelace loved stripes and sparkles on hers. Some people painted each nail a different color, while others celebrate holidays, like Valentine's Day, with an appropriate manicure motif. After five years of art school, Dyan Hill became a manicurist and perfected a rendering of a Chinese dragon in turquoise, gold, orange, lime green and fuchsia on one of singer Linda Miles' nails. Not to be outdone, manicurist Paula Johnson created a "full house" by depicting a "handful of cards" on a client's ten fingernails.

Most nail fads begin on the West Coast, where people are generally more receptive to experimental and even outlandish innovations. Veteran manicurist Minnie Smith, who pioneered acrylic extensions, has a clientele which includes Tina Sinatra, Linda Lovelace, Mitzi Gaynor and Leslie Uggams. These are people in show biz, where the motto is more often than not, "Anything extravagant and eyecatching goes!"

The nail-salon scene can provide a regular social event. Jessica Vartougian, who is now opening nail clinics across the country (newest in Bloomingdale's and Lord and Taylor in New York City) told me that since she has become a successful nail-salon mogul, what she misses most is the regular coffeeklatch of the stars that takes place among her "regulars" at her Beverly Hills salon.

"Nails by Nena" was the phrase once synonymous with nail wrapping in New York. Marriage transported Nena to Los

Angeles, and she now practices her craft in a very sedate Beverly Hills salon that accommodates one client at a time. Although her services have been employed for such special needs as augmenting Barbra Streisand's nails for *A Star Is Born* (not for breakage, but because Barbra usually wears her nails short on one hand so she can play the guitar), Nena caters to a basically conservative (by Los Angeles standards) clientele. However, one midnight Nena did receive a frantic call from a devoted client, who had just deplaned with a broken nail, begging for permission to arrive at Nena's residence for an emergency repair.

There are 83 nail salons listed in the Los Angeles Yellow Pages. Joan Rivers' cabaret, The Little Club, has just been converted into a nail emporium. Nails are becoming big business.

Grace's Nail Salon, in Beverly Hills, has about ten manicurists, five on each side of the room, working away on the hands of clients as diverse as the very rich, who schedule their appointments between tennis and the gym, and secretaries who enjoy their luxurious nails as their one luxury and status symbol.

All the manicurists who work at Grace's are trained by Grace at a cost to them of $400. The training is available only to those who have a license in cosmetology. Halfway through the special training, Grace observes their work and tells them if they are qualified, on the basis of talent or learning so far displayed, to work at Grace's Nail Salon. If you are given the royal nod, you may finish the course (500 hours) and earn the privilege of renting a chair in her salon.

There is much talk of "infidelity" among the various salons, like who really trained who, and then opened a shop down the street, who stole what procedure and called it their own, who is most "in" and really an artist, and who time has passed by.

Grace teaches her students the reason for every step of the manicure, "even why you hold the nail file at a certain angle."

I asked my manicurist what was the most outrageous thing anyone ever requested at the salon, having heard all the crazy tales of American flags, butterflies, gold initials, bicentennial motifs, etc. She blankly denied that any extraordinary request ever took place at Grace's. About ten minutes later a client entered the salon and took the booth next to us, loudly complaining that she had lost "still another diamond from her nail." It turns out that the shop sells diamonds (starting at $30) which can be glued into the nail. A jeweler's drill is used to make a hole in the nail plate (above the nail bed, of course), and the diamond is glued in place.

If the diamonds imbedded in the nail didn't strike her as the least bit outrageous, you will understand that gold nails ($35 a nail, $350 a set) are considered de rigueur in Los Angeles. A complete set of diamond-encrusted gold motifs were applied to a customer at Saks in Beverly Hills at a cost of $2,880.

MY HOLLYWOOD NAIL SPA MANICURE

Appointments are kept promptly at Grace's Nail Salon. The usual manicure here includes the nail wrap, or "Juliette" as this is called on the West Coast (cone-shaped fibrous mending tissues are glued to and wrapped under each nail). The manicure takes about an hour, but you should allow one-half hour extra, if possible, for drying. About halfway through my manicure at Grace's, my manicurist asked me if I wished to go to the bathroom. Since it has been years since anyone asked me that, I was amused to discover that the manicurists at Grace's are taught to pay attention to the "Three Ps," i.e., Payment, Potty and Parking (fishing out the client's car keys). She carefully wrapped each nail with mending paper, using a mixture of nail mender and Duco cement to smooth the papers down. Crazy Glue was carefully applied to only the inside of a small slit on one nail. She constantly dipped an orange stick into a large crystal brandy snifter containing polish remover, and used it to smooth and remove any excess anything. Silver baby porringers were used for lotions and "soaks." She used five coats of enamel in all—

two different base coats, specially chosen for my "case," two coats of colored enamel and a sealer. Colored enamel was applied to the underside of my nails. It was a terrific manicure, which surprisingly cost about a third less than in New York.

The Perfect Women's Manicure

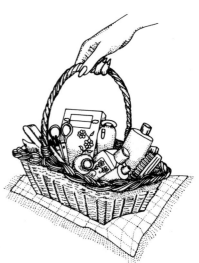

ℳANICURE ON A NIGHT when your required activities are about as vigorous as watching your favorite TV show. Really pamper yourself. Keep everything you need handy. I like a wooden basket with a handle (Easter basket style) to carry everything I need. This saves time and eliminates the excuse that you couldn't find all your "stuff." Ideally, after the manicure the nails should be left unpolished overnight. The experts say the rest from polish is good for the nails.

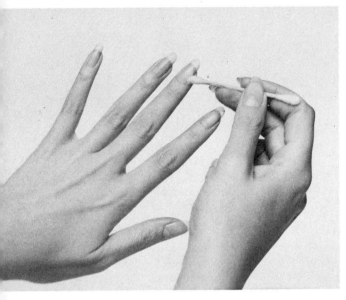

1. Use Q-Tip to remove hard-to-get polish

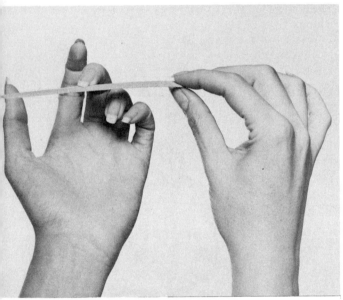

2. File methodically

1. Saturate a wad of cotton in polish remover and gently press it against the nail. Stroke from base to tip, keeping the liquid off the cuticle as much as possible. Then take a Q-Tip (or cotton-wrapped orange stick), dip in remover, and wipe off any remaining traces of enamel. Remember, this is a strong chemical, so wash it off your hands, and dry them thoroughly. Don't, however, soak them at this point, because the next project is filing, and you don't want softened nails, which are more prone to tears when any pressure is applied.

2. File with an emery board, holding the board flat against the edge of your nail. Don't saw. Just file in one direction towards the center. And remember, don't file too deeply at the sides.

3. Now give yourself one of the special treatments, like warm olive oil or honey (see Special Treats, page 179) and sit for a while with plastic gloves.

4. Apply cuticle cream to each nail.

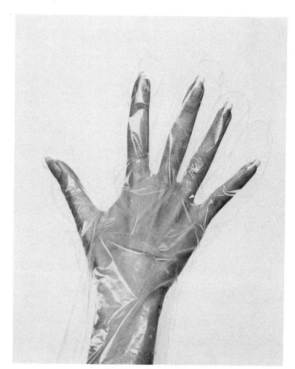

3. Use plastic gloves for an olive oil treat

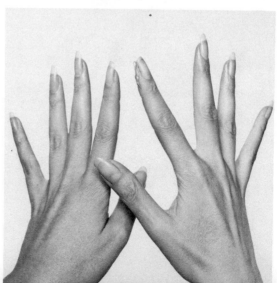

4. Apply cuticle cream

5. Soak in dishwashing liquid and warm water for about ten minutes. This procedure softens the cuticle, loosens any dirt lodged under and around the nail, and removes any little filing bits that might still be on your nails.

6. Use your soft nailbrush to scrub your nails, as well as the skin on your hands. Do this gently and any dead dried skin will fall away.

7. Now use a pumice stone or stick to soften rough edges

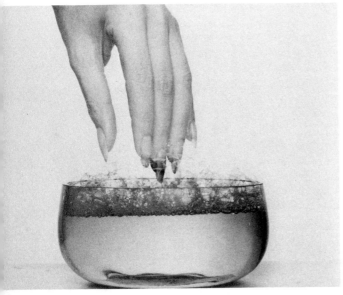

5. Dishwashing-liquid soak

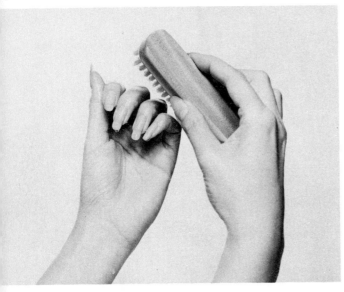

6. Use a soft nail brush

around your nails and to aid in removing any stains on the fingers. Dry hands and gently push back the cuticle at the base of your nails with a nubby washcloth that you launder regularly. This would be the ideal time to use a scrub or mask described on page 180, because removal of dead surface skin facilitates the absorption of hand lotion or cream.

8. If you choose to use liquid cuticle remover, apply and gently push back the cuticle with a cotton-wrapped orange stick.

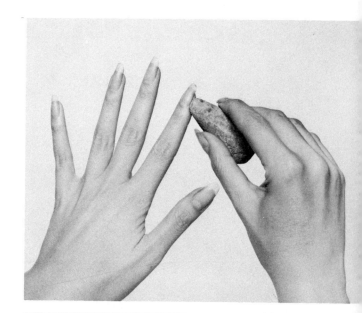

7. Pumice rough edges

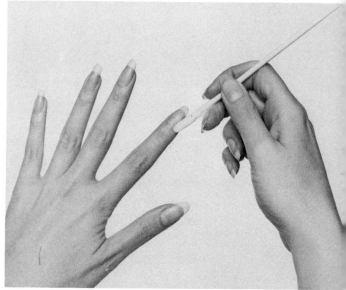

8. Push cuticles back with cotton-wrapped orange stick

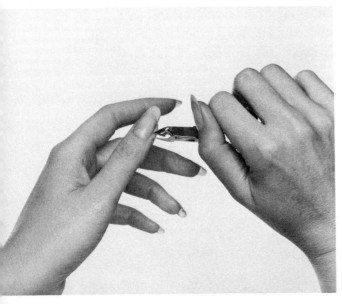

9. Clip cuticles if necessary

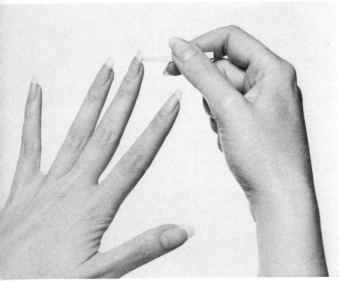

10. Clean undernail with Stim-U-Dents

9. Cut any raggedy edges and hangnails. Do not cut the rim at the base of your nail, as it is there to protect new nail growth. Rinse off cuticle remover. *Note:* This is a strong chemical and should not be left on the nail or cuticle for any length of time.

10. Clean under nails with cotton-wrapped orange stick or Stim-U-Dent (little wooden sticks sold for dental cleaning, which soften when moistened). For stubborn stains, dip the wrapped orange stick or Stim-U-Dent in hydrogen peroxide (or even Clorox if necessary). Rinse off.

11. Buff nails to improve circulation and smooth the appearance of the nail's surface. Buff in one direction only to prevent the nail from getting too hot. Special polishing paste, which is like jeweler's polish, is sold in most drug and department stores and can be used with the buffer to achieve a nice shine. Do not use a buffing paste if you are going to use enamel on your nails, as it reduces the "grip" on the nails' surface for the enamel to properly adhere, and can encourage early chipping. Repair any breaks or tears now (see Professional Repair for Broken and Split Nails, p. 105). Leave your nails "bare" overnight, at this point, if possible, to let them rest.

12. Select your base coat, enamel color and sealer before beginning application, so that you won't risk smudges while

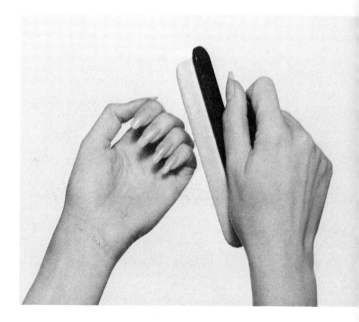

11. Buff in one direction

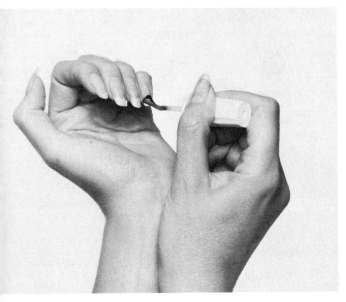

12. Apply base coat

your nails are drying. Start with a base coat, which is essential if you are going to use colored enamel. The following is the best procedure for applying base coats and enamels: Dip in the brush and revolve the tip inside the neck of the bottle to remove most of the polish. As you apply the brush to the nail, the polish in the upper part of the bristles will flow down evenly. Keep turning the brush as you go. Use the corner of the brush around the edges. (If you are right-handed, apply polish to your left hand first.)

13. After vigorously shaking the closed bottle of nail enamel, roll the bottle between your palms for a few seconds to further ensure that the temperature of the enamel will be warm and therefore easiest to apply. Some people like the support of a hard surface for steadiness of application. I seem to do better with holding my nails folded toward my palms, as in the picture. This is probably because I am nearsighted.

14. Use matches to clean up any polish that has spilled on to the sides of the fingers. Use a matchbook with hard edges to

remove any small smears from the sides of the nails—this often eliminates excessive use of polish remover around the cuticles. Do not smoke or strike matches during this stage of your manicure.

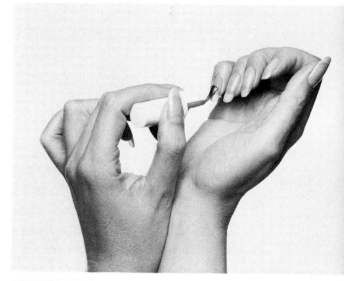

13. Apply polish

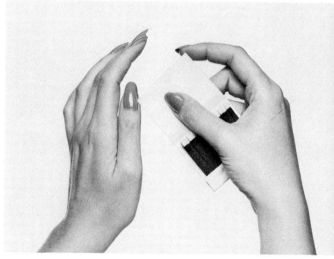

14. Matchbook cleaning

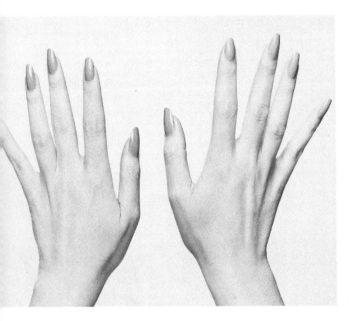

15. The manicured hand

15. Apply two coats of enamel and let your nails dry thoroughly between coats. This step is as important with colorless as with colored enamel, because the enamel is protecting and strengthening your nail surface. Pale-pink polishes sometimes require three coats of polish to prevent a streaked look. Finish with a sealer (which can sometimes be the same product as your base coat). Let dry as long as you can. A good test for tackiness is to lightly touch your tongue to your nails. If the nail doesn't taste of polish, it's dry.

The Perfect Men's Manicure

1. Remove any enamel, if you wear it, with a cotton ball saturated with polish remover. File the edge of your nail at a 45-degree angle. Hold the board (or metal nail file) flat against the edge of your nail. File in one direction toward the center. Avoid painful hangnails by not filing too deeply at the sides. Ideally, men's nails should show a "hair" of white nail extending ¼ inch beyond the fingertip.

1. File

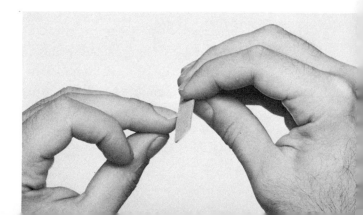

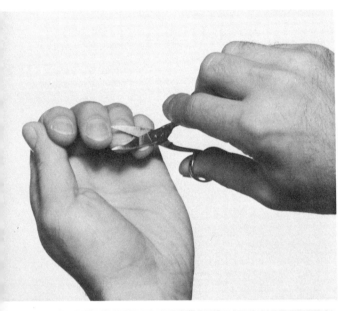

2. Trim

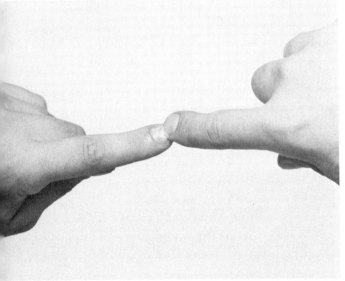

3. Apply cuticle cream

2. If you prefer, you can cut your nails with manicuring scissors. While not as precise as filing, cutting is a faster procedure (and the risk of tearing a nail with nail scissors is minimal, as most men have short nails).

3. Apply a small amount of cuticle cream to each nail.

4. Soak in dishwashing liquid and warm water for about ten minutes, if possible. This softens the cuticle, loosens any dirt lodged under and around the nail, and removes any little filing particles that might still be on your nails.

5. Use a soft nailbrush to scrub your nails as well as the skin on your hands.

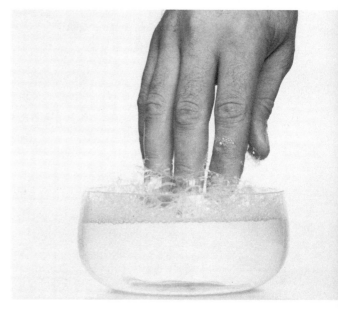

4. Soak

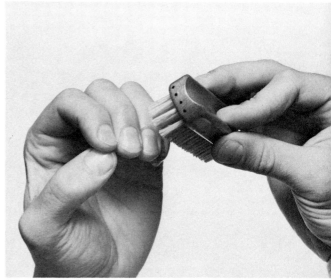

5. Brush

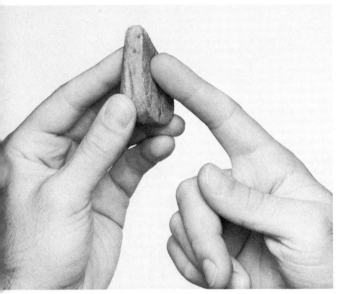

6. Pumice

6. A pumice stone moistened in the warm water can soften rough edges around your fingernails as well as any calluses on your palms and fingers. Pumice also removes most stains that don't respond to regular soap and water or the rubbing of a lemon wedge over the discolored area.

7. Dry hands thoroughly and gently push back the cuticle at the base of your nails with a nubby washcloth that you launder regularly. If you prefer cuticle remover to the cream (many men do, as it is faster, although a harsher chemical) apply at this

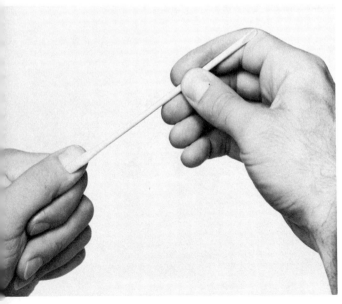

7. Push back cuticles

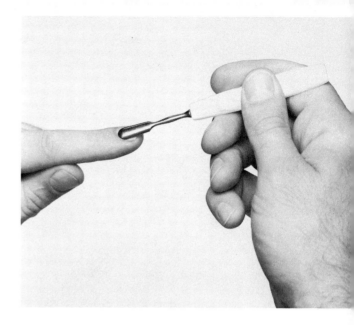

8. Metal cuticle pusher

point and gently push back the cuticle with a cotton-wrapped orange stick.

8. A metal cuticle pusher can be used, but take care to be gentle with this implement, as the cuticle rim at the base of the nail is delicate and is there to protect the nail bed.

9. Cut any ragged cuticles and hangnails with a cuticle scissors or trimmers, but do not cut the cuticle flap that protects the nail bed. Wash off any cuticle remover from the nail, as this is a strong chemical and should not be left on the nails.

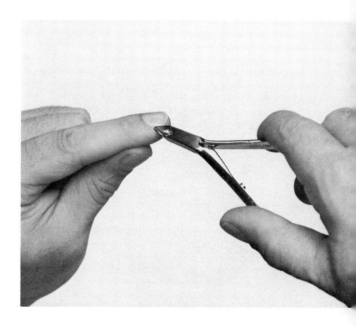

9. Cut cuticles

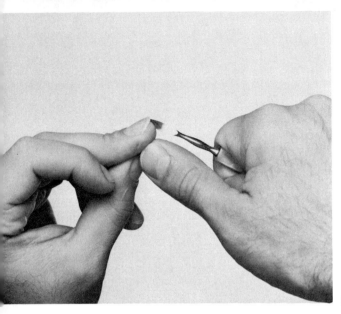

10. Clean under nails

10. Clean under the nail with an orange stick, a metal implement designed for this purpose, or Stim-U-Dents (little wooden sticks used mainly for dental cleaning, which soften when moistened. For stubborn stains or dirt that has remained imbedded under the nail for some time, dip the cotton-wrapped stick or Stim-U-Dent in hydrogen peroxide, or even Clorox, if necessary. Rinse off.

11. Apply hand lotion at this stage, if desired.

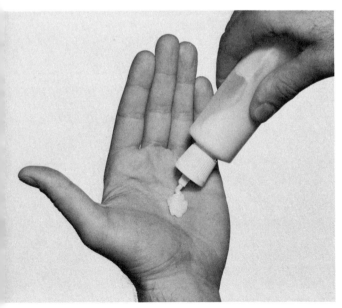

11. Apply hand lotion

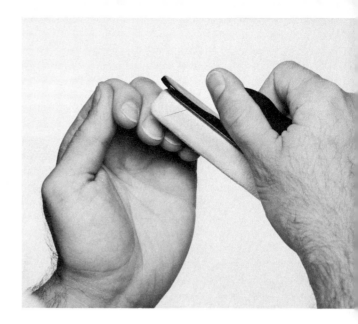

12. Buff

12. Buff nails to improve circulation and smooth the appearance of the nail's surface. Buff in one direction only to prevent the nail from getting too hot. Special polishing paste, which is like jeweler's polish, is sold in most drug and department stores, and can be used with the buffer to achieve a nice shine.

13. Some men like to use a light coat of colorless enamel. Before applying, at this last stage, remove any traces of cream and/or lotion from the nails. I have discovered a special original

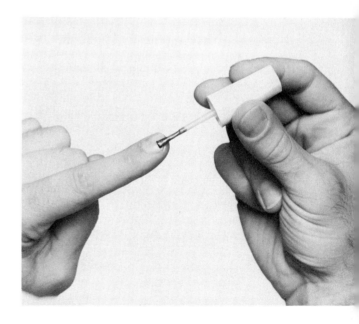

13. Apply enamel or base

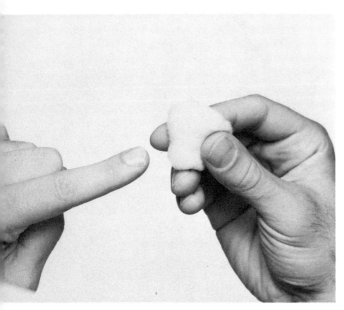

14. Wipe off frosted base

process for improving the appearance of men's nails without the high gloss of enamel: Apply a coat of frosted base coat to the nail.

14. Then quickly wipe over the nail surface with a cotton swab. The result is a surprisingly white, clean look that is more natural than clear polish.

The Health and Happiness
of Your Hands

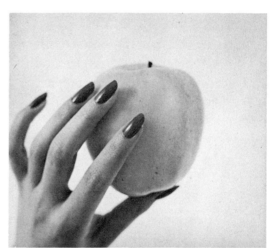

ꟻINGERNAILS are like mirrors, reflecting information when the body suffers disease, infection or severe dietary deficiency. New York internist Dr. Bry Benjamin told me that doctors often watch the nails carefully during an operation. If the nail pales, or takes on a bluish tinge, it could be a sign of dropping blood pressure or an early state of shock.

DIAGNOSIS BY THE HANDS

These diseases can often be detected by changes in the hands and/or nails:

> *Mongolism*—a short fifth finger.
> *Sickle cell disease and congenital high or low blood pressure*—spiderlike fingers.
> *Endocarditis*—hemorrhaging under the nail.
> *Psoriasis*—pitted, thickened nails, sometimes separated from the nail bed.
> *Addison's disease*—discoloration of the skin.
> *Thyroid disease*—puffiness.
> *Lung disease*—hardening of the skin, club-shaped nails. These are the result of low oxygen levels, and are also found in people who have congenital heart disease, as well as those who live at high altitudes—who also have lowered oxygen levels.

Of course, some conditions apply only to the hands, and are "topical," like bacteria and fungi, chemical irritations and conditions caused by accidents.

HANDICAPS

Arthritis, which is hereditary, usually on the female side, is treated with exercises (like squeezing a rubber ball) and paraffin baths, which give deep heat. Palsy, or shaking, is often relieved by tranquilizing drugs, like Valium. Surprisingly, rehabilitation of the hands of stroke victims involves improvement of muscular connection, rather than coordination. There are, in fact, surgeons who specialize in hands, like Lee Ramsay Straub. After a stroke or severe arthritis, the fingers may be locked in an awkward position, and operative procedures can improve both dexterity and appearance.

•

Slam Stewart, one of the most famous jazz bass players, has enormous hands, which he considers an advantage because they give him an increased reach. Having suffered a stroke, which must be a musician's nightmare, Stewart told me that miraculously he was playing again in a month or two. "Although my action hand was strong enough, I had more feeling first in my left hand, which is my fingering hand."

DETERGENT HANDS

People who keep their hands in water a lot, or in any moist environment, give bacteria and fungi an opportunity to thrive. The backs of the hands become red and sensitive. The tissue at the sides of the nail can become inflamed (called paronychia). Keep the hands dry until the condition is better and treat with creams and lotions to prevent further surface moisture loss. Gloves may seem inconvenient, especially to men, but they arrest the problem and prompt a fast recovery.

SWEATY PALMS

There are two types of sweat glands in our skin: apocrine and eccrine. Most sweat glands are eccrine; these glands are tubular coils based in the middle layer of the skin, and are over almost all parts of the body. The pores are formed as each gland reaches up through the skin's top layer and excretes a thin, clear, watery liquid, which we call perspiration, or sweat.

Although we perspire more in warm weather, we can experience damp palms from nervous tension, anxieties and sexual stimulation. Patients often consult doctors to complain of constant sweaty palms. (*Note:* Although there is no known medical cure, hypnosis has been effective in curing some chronic cases of sweaty palms.)

•

NO SWEAT

"Although I have to take precautions with my hands like carrying my guitar case with the left hand, never with the hand that does the plucking, surprisingly, sweat is never a factor in my playing. Even in conditions of extreme heat or tension, I don't sweat. I have dry hands. If I didn't, I'd be changing my strings all night!"

—Guitarist BUCKY PIZZARELLI

•

THREE OLD WIVES' TALES REFUTED

1. A cut in the piece of skin that connects the thumb to the rest of the hand does not cause dire consequences (like fainting or bleeding to death)! It just hurts like any other cut.

2. Knuckle cracking does not lead to enlarged or distorted joints.

3. While the size of one's hands is often in direct proportion to the size of one's feet, any relationship to the size of the male genitalia has thus far not been statistically correlated.

SIZE OF HANDS

While the size of a golfer's hand is no indication of his proficiency, the size of Wilt Chamberlain's hand is probably as important to his success as his height. Ironically, Super Bowl star Lynn Swann, wide receiver for the Pittsburgh Steelers, has, by his own evaluation "hands much smaller than the average player."

THE HAND GYM OR "HAND SPRINGS"

The hand gym was developed by Dr. Semyon Krewer, a nuclear physicist, to help cure his own rheumatoid arthritis. Designed originally to help hands affected by disease or surgery regain strength and flexibility, the hand gym is now being used by guitarists, pianists, sportsmen, dentists and others who are interested in attaining maximum strength, flexibility and dexterity of their hands and fingers. Finger and thumb workouts are accomplished by means of exercise bars, foam cushions and elastic bands. The hand gym is a clear plastic triangular seven by seven by seven-inch form, soon to be on display at the Museum of Modern Art. At present it is available at surgical-supply houses and some drug stores and costs $20.

THE HAND HAZARDS OF
BEING A MUSICIAN

Jazz pianist Marian McPartland: "At one time Lloyds of London insured my hands. It seems that I had this horrible fantasy of someone ice-skating over my hands. But then I don't skate much, so I dropped the policy. Actually, the only injury I ever had was when I broke my wrist in a Jeep accident in Nuremberg on the way to the trials. Soon after, upon arrival in the U.S., Jimmy [her then husband, jazz trumpeter, Jimmy McPartland] took me right over to Eddie Condon's jazz club, which I had been hearing about for years. I was so excited to be there that I played with my fingers sticking out of the cast."

Drummer Bob Rosengarten: "I take care not to get bone bruises. Playing the bongos and congas, I've had a few. Actually, drums are highly varnished and you can't play with any pressure for too long, although some rock drummers do. After twenty-five years of playing the drums as a married person, I decided to remove my wedding ring while playing in order to avoid any possible injury to my fingers. After suffering a sprained wrist playing volleyball, I now stick to water sports."

When he was fourteen, internationally famous conductor Seiji Ozawa, having already begun a musical career as a pianist, broke his two index fingers playing rugby. "I thought I would have to give up music. I thought of composing. Then my teacher said "Why not conducting?" And in so doing, turned an injury into a profitable career direction.

TURNING BACK THE HANDS OF TIME

Compared to facial skin, the skin on the backs of the hands is thin and has few oil glands. It takes more wear and tear, dries up easily, and there is little flesh underneath the skin to support moisture. Also, hands get more exposure to the elements than we realize. If you have left the beach to do some shopping, you may not be facing the sun, but your hands may still be sunbathing. According to New York dermatologist Norman Orentreich, women's hands age earlier than men's; and the hands of Caucasians age earlier than those of blacks and Eurasians. Dr. Orentreich, one of the first doctors to successfully use silicone injections to smooth out facial wrinkles, is now using the same procedure to plump out the skin on hands that have wrinkled with age and/or excessive exposure. Dr. Orentreich stressed, however, that this is a highly specialized procedure. Very small amounts (1/50 to 1/80 cc.) of 100 percent pure silicone are injected into the skin. The treatments are spread out over six-week intervals to allow new collagen deposits to develop around the droplets of skin cells. Each visit costs $75; a complete series runs about $1500 and obviously takes some time. While costly, this is really good news for people with prematurely aging skin on their hands (especially those who have had facial surgery, but are experiencing "hand lag"). Just please check with your local medical authorities before you go shopping for this RX.

LIVER SPOTS

These discolorations, which look somewhat like freckles, can show up any time after age thirty, and actually have nothing whatsoever to do with the liver. They are caused by aging and exposure to the sun. A paste of salt and lemon juice can sometimes cause a satisfactory fading of the spots. Over-the-counter products are sold to "erase" them. These products contain the active ingredient hydroquinone, which is a bleaching agent accepted by the FDA. They also contain an abrasive, or mild sloughing agent. The best-selling one is Esoterica.

Dr. Orentreich is now using two procedures to remove so-called "liver spots." Desiccation is a method of burning off the spot electrically. A scab is instantly formed, which falls off the skin in about a week. A red spot remains for about another week, after which the surface is clear. The actual administration of the electrical current can be mildly uncomfortable if the spots are large or numerous. In such cases, cryosurgery is indicated. This involves touching the spots with a solid stick of freezing carbon dioxide. This method is relatively painless but takes a longer period of time to completely heal. Both methods cost about $75 and are done in the doctor's office.

DERMABRASION

This method of removing pigmentation from skin is not generally approved for use on the backs of your hands as it can seriously rob the skin of its natural moisture, which would speed the aging process. Beware of any salon that offers this service to remove liver spots. Reputable doctors use dermabrasions on the hands only to remove a since-regretted tattoo.

The Nail File

What are nails? Nails are specialized outgrowths of skin tissue that enable us to use our fingers more effectively. The nail protects the hypersensitive nerve endings below the nail and on the fingertips. (We all know that "Cut to the quick" means "Ouch!") The nail, much like hair, is mostly proteins, with small amounts of calcium, phosphorous and trace metals. Also, like the hair, most of the nail is made of layers of dead cells held together with tiny quantities of moisture and fat. The moisture and fat decrease with age, which is why nails peel more as we get older. The live, growing portion of the nail (the matrix) is at the edge of the cuticle and just behind it.

What affects nail growth? Nails generally take six months

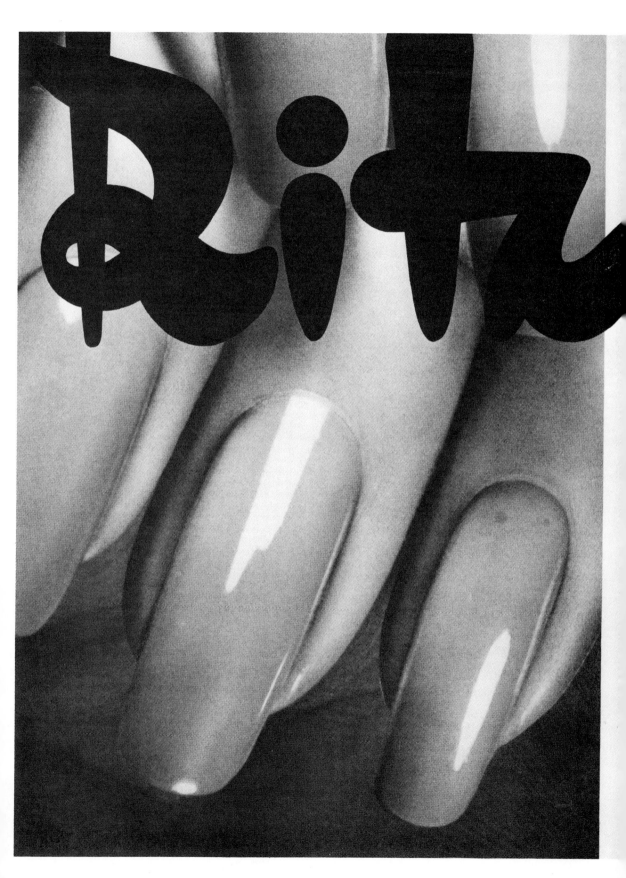

to fully grow out. They grow faster in childhood (but stop during childhood diseases), and slow down at about age twenty-five. Nails grow fastest in hot weather, with increased metabolism, and slowest in winter, when they also become more brittle. They speed along during pregnancy, but slow down during periods of serious illness, nervous shock and even viral infections. The thumbnail grows the slowest, while the nail of the middle finger seems to grow the fastest, as do all the nails on the hand you use the most. Nails thicken with age, but activities like typing, buffing, piano playing and nail biting (!) make them grow faster. Contrary to popular opinion, nails do not continue to grow after death. It just looks that way because the surrounding skin tissue shrinks.

NAIL PROBLEMS

White spots and ridges: These can be caused by a blow or too much pressure at the base of the nail. They will eventually grow out, as they don't involve damage to the nail bed.

Little white flecks: These little markings on the nail can be caused by a trauma, small or large. They will grow out in six months.

Yellowing can be the result of chemicals and dyes in household and gardening products, leaks from colored nail enamel (especially with failure to use a base coat), and prolonged use of antibiotics like tetracycline.

Excessive breaking and peeling: Check for possible excessive exposure to detergents, metal cleansers and other household products. Also beware of the possibility of damage from damp inner surface of rubber gloves. (These gloves should always be dry, and should be removed frequently.) Use creams or a good olive oil soak (see "Treats," page 179).

Hangnails: These start with splits in or near the cuticle. Hangnails are actually ragged flaps of dead skin. Not only are they uncomfortable, but they can become infected. Don't pull them off. Cut them with a sharp scissors and use cuticle cream to keep the skin soft.

Accidents: A sudden blow from a hammer, or a finger being caught in a door can cause the area of the nail to bleed and a black spot of coagulated blood may appear. Apply something cold quickly and elevate the hand to prevent an unnecessary accumulation of blood. The spot will grow out if the damage was not done at the base (matrix, or growing portion) of the nail. A more serious injury can cause the nail to loosen or even shed. The best RX is to see a doctor, who may have to drill a hole through the nail plate to let the blood drain. This hole is not permanent, however, and will grow out with the nail.

SEPARATION OF THE NAIL FROM THE BED

Technically called "onycholysis," this separation can be caused by psoriasis, iron deficiency, thyroid disease or injury. More often, however, it is caused by allergies or fungus infection. Dermatologists are finding more of these conditions with the increased popularity of acrylic powders used in some nail salons and sold in some "nail-extension" kits. However, a "Saran Wrap" effect can occur, softening the nail. Doctors may prescribe topical and internal medications to alleviate the condition.

NAILS AND DIET

Should you take gelatin to add inches to your nails? No, unless you are interested in adding pounds of flesh to your hips. Doctors simply advocate a "healthy, well-balanced" diet for healthy nails. However, deficiencies can lead to the following:

Dry, brittle nails: Vitamin A and calcium deficiencies.

Fragile nails with horizontal and vertical ridges: Vitamin B deficiency.

Opaque white bands: Possible shortage of protein, Vitamin A, calcium or iron.

Cracking and splitting: Riboflavin, Vitamin B_2 deficiency.

Concave nail: Iron deficiency.

White spots: May be lack of zinc (but more likely a blow or small trauma).

Dry, hardened cuticle: Perhaps from antibiotics.

Soaps, Lotions and Other Tools of the Trade

ACCORDING TO REVLON research experts, the products you use on your hands, such as creams, lotions and nail products, are tested more rigorously than the food products that are permitted to be sold on our supermarket shelves. Hand products are not only carefully tested for possible allergic reaction, but also subjected to extremes of temperature (freezing, hours of baking in ovens), simulating all possible environmental conditions.

You may still find chemicals in the products that don't agree with your own skin or nails. Fortunately, since the Fair Packaging Act, ingredients are listed on the package so you can check what you are buying, as well as what you may be sensitive

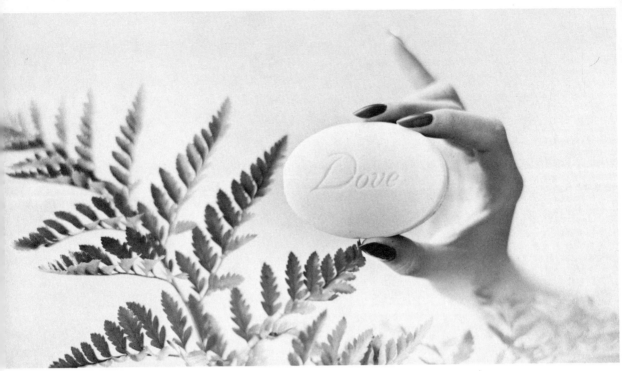

JOE LONG

to. Also, if the ingredients are not listed on the package, you have a clue as to how long the product has been sitting on the store shelf.

Note the weight of the product listed on the label. Shapes of bottles can be deceptive. The shape of the bottle may also indicate its usefulness to you: I find some bottles of nail polish beautiful but very difficult to handle. Some nail-polish brushes are easier to use than others. A lotion that costs a little more because it has a pump dispenser may be worth it for the convenience. And don't discount the psychological bonus of anything you buy: it may be worth it to you to pay extra for a lotion that makes you feel elegant, a new nail color that makes you feel in vogue, or even a soap that tells you that you are treating yourself better than you ever have before.

SOAP

Soap is not only the most obvious but also the most basic beauty and health aid for both men and women. Dirt, if allowed to dry in the crevices of the skin and around the nails, seems to do instant and observable damage. Clean is better. Any mild soap will do. And it can be as thrifty as a supermarket variety, as special as Basis or Clinique, or as sensually pleasing as one of the elegantly scented soaps made from expensive perfumes. Get one you like and use it.

NAIL BRUSHES

These vary from inexpensive plastic brushes from the five and ten to the fine and costly English bristle ones sold at good drug and department stores. Make sure that your brush is relatively soft so as not to tear the cuticle or separate the nail from the nail bed at the "quick." Nail brushes clean and massage the nails nicely if used with a gentle touch.

SLOUGHING AGENTS

These are creams or pastes that contain mild abrasives or astringent liquids, which remove any dead skin, allowing the remaining skin surface more readily to accept the softening effect of a really rich cream or lotion. These sloughing agents also help to remove stains. You can buy creams that contain especially fine pumice or oatmeal. You can also check at local health-food stores for combinations you can make yourself. I use Clinique Cleansing Lotion II, which is a product manufactured as a facial toner. I saturate cotton and carefully go over the backs of my hands and cuticles. The cotton looks shockingly dirty by the time I'm finished. Then I follow up immediately with application of a super-rich face cream such as Orlane's Creme Astral or Arden's Visible Difference. The result is soft and luxurious (and hands that can stand the careful scrutiny of the closeup camera).

HAND LOTIONS

Hand lotions are basically oil (vegetable or mineral), water, fragrance, and emulsifying agents that bind them together. The purpose of a hand lotion is to replace the moisture lost in the hand and leave a thin film of emollient between the skin surface and the air to retard moisture from evaporating. Lotions can curb chapping, dryness and skin irritations and make the skin feel soft. Technically the lotions don't actually "heal" but rather replace the lost moisture until the skin condition is better. They can also make your hands smell delicious, like almonds or crushed flowers, or other fragrances that can turn you, or the person you are with, on.

Choose a lotion with easy-to-apply features, like a pump handle, and use it as often as you can. You can buy several pump-applicator plastic bottles in a small size to keep in the kitchen, bathroom, bedside, the car.

The giant size Vaseline Intensive Care is a real value. Buy big and have your favorite lotion in nice little plastic pump or squeeze bottles wherever you need it. The name "Intensive Care" was chosen because the lotion was developed during the time of the Vietnam war, when the term "intensive care unit" came into use (to be further popularized by the movie and subsequent TV show *M.A.S.H.*), to indicate emergency aid for severe physical problems.

EMERY BOARDS AND NAIL FILES

Emery boards smooth rough nail edges and trim and shape the nail. They come in a 7-inch professional size and a 4½-inch pocket size. One side of the board has a heavier grain to finish the nail and smooth any rough pieces of skin that have hardened at the edges of the fingertips.

Some professional manicurists swear by Diamond Dust metal files. I prefer emery boards because they are more flexible.

However, metal files are great to carry in your purse because they don't fall apart if exposed to moisture (as emery boards can). Famous manicurist Nena Ricco also advises using a metal file to open jewelry, thus saving stress on the nails.

File your nails only when they are hard and dry. Never file after you've soaked your nails or just had a bath. Hold the board or file flat against the edge of the nail at a 45-degree angle. Stay away from corners (where breaks most often start). And don't saw. File in one direction; your nail is like many layers of paper, and sawing back and forth with a file or board will cause it to peel and chip.

•

Primitives used to file their nails with shells that had a sprinkling of sand applied with fish glue.

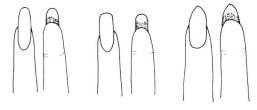

NAIL SHAPES

Your best guide for a nail shape is the cuticle, which rims the base of the nail, or "moon," if it shows. It is oval and an oval shape is ideal for maximum protection and use of the nail. It is also the classic shape for nails.

Special Tip: To be assured of a perfectly shaped nail, check it out from the palm side. The shape of the nail should look even from front and back.

Square tips are "in" for now, and look okay if your fingers are slim. Pointed nails give heavy hands the illusion of tapered fingers. Very pointed nails just look silly and break too easily. If you are into a "dangerous woman" look, you might want to risk them, although guys often tell me that these nails are a general turnoff.

Men's nails should show just a bit of white tip. It was once thought that ideally a woman's nail should extend ¼ inch beyond the fingertip, although today anything goes.

NAIL SCISSORS

Some manicurists use scissors if they are going to cut the length of the nail considerably. I prefer filing. In any case, don't use scissors on soft, wet nails, as the nail may easily break farther down on the nail bed than you intended. And use scissors only for reducing the length, not shaping.

NAIL CLIPPERS

Save nail clippers for your toenails. They can tear your fingernail and create raggedy edges.

REMOVERS

For those who wear nail polish, clear as well as colored, remover is essential. This applies to men as well as women. Peeling off polish with your nails (or teeth!) removes an important layer of natural moisture and can also take off a layer of nail.

Nail-polish removers have various descriptive subtitles, such as "non-smear," "with oil," "gentle," etcetera. You can also buy remover pads encased in foil, which are relatively expensive but great if you're traveling. Removers are usually a combination of one or more organic solvents (often acetone), water, oil (to minimize the drying effect of the solvent) and a fragrance (to mask any harsh odor). Prices vary, and it is wise to check the amounts on the label of the bottle. A wide selection is available. If fragrance and skin sensitivity are important to you, as they are to me, you may have to pay a little more for the one you want.

Never soak your nails in remover. To use a remover properly, saturate a wad or ball of cotton with remover and press it gently against the nail plate. Stroke the polish off gently. Then take a Q-Tip, dip in remover and wipe off whatever bits of polish are still on your nails. Removers contain some strong chemicals, so wash it off your hands immediately.

Ideally, at this point, you would apply some softening cream, and let your hands "rest" overnight with a moisture treat before applying new polish the next day.

Special safety note: These products are extremely flammable. Do not use near flame. And do not smoke while using them!

CUTICLE CREAM

My favorite cuticle cream is Dior's Creme Abricot, but plain petroleum jelly works well. Apply before soaking your hands. After soaking, gently push back the cuticle with a towel or orange stick. This helps to create a natural oval shape to the nail. Dr. Earl Brauer, of Revlon research, likened the cuticle at the end of the nail to a fine watch crystal. It protects the nail matrix and should never be removed. Cuticle cream performs softening miracles if left on overnight.

CUTICLE REMOVER

As your nail grows, some cuticle naturally remains on the nail plate. While a cuticle cream softens, a cuticle remover dissolves this skin. It should be washed off your hands after use.

ORANGEWOOD STICKS

Orangewood sticks are pointed at one end for cleaning under your nails, and flat at the other end for pushing the cuticle gently away from the nail plate (after soaking and creaming). You can wrap cotton on the pointed end and dip it in the polish remover to clean smeared polish on the cuticle.

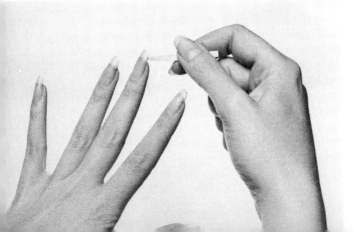

CUTICLE CLIPPERS AND TRIMMERS

Use cuticle clippers on ragged sides or hangnails *only*. Don't ever use them to cut the cuticle flap that protects the nail bed. (Use creams and removers with care and you'll be rewarded with healthier-looking nails.) If the skin on the sides of the nail is tough, soften the skin with a pumice stone soaked in soapy water, or the smooth side of an emery board. Needless to say, don't use your teeth or nails as a substitute cuticle clipper!

PUMICE STONE OR STICK

Not only are these wonderful for softening cuticles on the sides of your nails, but they also help remove stains from your hands. Soak the stone or stick in soapy water first to do the best and safest job.

STIM-U-DENTS

These soft wooden toothpicklike sticks, sold at drugstores for cleaning the teeth, are also great for removing dirt from the sides of nails. Dampened, Stim-U-Dents are pliable but strong. Because of their flexibility they are preferable to metal or orangewood sticks. I also use them dipped in hydrogen peroxide (or Clorox for extreme problems) to remove stubborn discolorations under the sides and top of the nail.

BUFFERS

Buffers can increase the stimulation of the nail bed under the plate, create a shiny surface, and reduce yellowing. Sizes range from 4¾ inches to 8 inches long; the buffer pad is covered with a chamois cloth which can sometimes be replaced. Dry buffing polish (a powder) can be applied to the chamois, whereas wet polish (paste) should be applied directly to the nails, and then buffed. Buff the nails in only one direction to prevent the nail from getting too hot.

Go easy, as buffing removes some of the natural oil or moisture from the nail surface. For shiny bare nails, use buffer paste and polish regularly.

There are kits available (like "P" Shine and Jovan) that contain emery boards with foam rubber sandwiched in between. These are used to sand down the surface of the nail and remove any ridges. The nail ridges will reappear as the nail grows out, so be careful that, when you smooth out the new growth, you don't sand the same surface again. These kits also contain moist pastes to buff onto the nail and shiny polishes to give a mirror finish.

WHITE PENCIL

The white pencil works as makeup when you have sheer, clear or no polish on your nails. It "colors" the exposed nail length by application to the underside of the nail. Moisten the point first. Apply only to clean nails, and be gentle near the quick. Wash off the excess. Don't use the plastic cap on the pencil as a nail cleaner; it is not pointed enough and is too stiff to be absolutely safe.

ELECTRIC MANICURE SETS

These manicure sets, electric or battery operated (Clairol makes a nice one), are excellent for those who are less than ambidextrous. They contain attachments for filing, callus remover, cuticle pusher, cuticle brush and buffer. Just watch what you are doing (especially with the file); they work so effortlessly, that you can do more work than you intend. Such a set is not essential, but just really nice to have. It makes a great gift.

HAND MAKEUP

Hand makeup covers scarred, discolored or severely reddened hands. It acts also as a good screen, which is a wise consideration for all of us, as we are rarely conscious of how often our hands are exposed to the sun. Just make sure it's waterproof.

NAIL ENAMELS

Base Coat

Base is a primer coat that smooths and protects the surface of the nail and enables the coat of colored enamel to bind better. Some nail lacquers can "bleed" into the nail plate, changing the color of the nail. While this is not serious, it is also not desirable. The "base" step is often eliminated by people who use colored polish. Popular hand models who change polish so often that they never worry about durability are tempted to skip this step too. But if they do, they may be put at a great disadvantage when a photo or commercial requires bare nails or clear polish; the nail plate that hasn't been protected habitually with a base coat doesn't glow with pink health; rather, it appears yellowed.

I like a base coat that contains some frosted enamel. It seems to give my nails maximum protection, and if I choose not to wear a colored enamel, the frosted base provides a nice finish. I would rather use two coats of a frosted base than a clear polish. Two coats of a frosted base under any enamel is my favorite way to smooth, prime and protect my nails, especially if I am using a red or dark enamel color. Chips are more noticeable and color bleeding is more apparent with the deeper shades, so I need maximum durability.

Nail Hardeners

Actually, all nail enamels are nail hardeners. The new products now being marketed as nail hardeners are colorless and contain nylon fibers to create a mesh effect on the nail. This coating is harder than regular enamel, but often doesn't produce as smooth a surface as regular enamels do. Nail hardeners occasionally contain formaldehyde, which can be damaging to the nail plate. Check the ingredients before you buy one of these.

Colored Enamel

Every season the cosmetics industry tries to entice us with new fashion colors without which life won't be worth living. I think this is terrific because it is one of the cheapest ways to feel *au courant*—even cheaper than most lipsticks!

To choose the best brand for you, note the shape of the bottle. Some polishes that have a "plume" on the brush are easy to apply. Some bottles tend to tip over when the brush is re-dipped. Some companies manufacture better applicator brushes than others (one little hair extending beyond the others is maddening when you are applying a colored polish to your nail).

Note: Colored enamel on your nails often masks dirt under your nail, so if you wear it, make doubly sure that you are cleaning the underneath portion of your nails.

Color Choice

What color should you use? Anything that turns you on. And don't stop there. You can mix several shades to create one that will be your personal trademark. Olive skin generally looks wonderful with coral and apricot shades, and not so good with pinks and lavenders; the latter enhance fair skins. I find that frosted polish wears better, in general, than cream, and looks great with a tan. You can also disguise the shape of your nails by the clever choice of polish, as well as how you apply that polish.

Short, wide fingers: Avoid intense shades; light colors are best for short nails or those which are growing out. Create an almond-shaped nail and leave a slight edge uncolored at each side to create a longer nail look.

Large-boned hands: The longer your nails, the slimmer your hands will look. Pale or "natural" polish plays down the size of the hand.

Extra-thin nails on wide fingers: Keep length fairly short, and again, choose a fairly neutral shade to blend in with the flesh tones.

FOR MAXIMUM USE
OF YOUR BOTTLE OF ENAMEL

1. If color separation occurs, shake the bottle vigorously.
2. Wipe the neck of the bottle after use, so enamel doesn't accumulate there. Close the bottle tightly so enamel doesn't

thicken, and also to permit you to reopen the bottle easily. If your polish does thicken, add a drop or two of enamel solvent, replace the bottle cap and shake vigorously. If polish still isn't thin enough, repeat the procedure till it glides on your nail smoothly. This solvent is sold where you buy your polish, but rarely displayed. It can prolong the life of a bottle of polish for ages. (Solvent can also help if you have used too much polish on a nail. Dip a cotton-wrapped orange stick in a solvent and brush lightly over the polish.)

3. Store enamel away from light and heat to prevent change in color and viscosity.

4. Enamels and solvents are inflammable, so do not use near any flame or while smoking.

Roll brush clockwise against neck of bottle

SEALERS

These are like the wax finish you apply to your perfectly adorned surface. Fabergé's nail glacé is terrific, and better than an additional coat of enamel because it is thinner.

DRYING OILS AND SPRAYS

These products are useful if you haven't left enough time for your manicure to dry properly. Weather watch: Humid and rainy weather can make thorough drying of nail polish take forever.

Adornments

*T*HE PAPAL RING, the British Royal Crown jewels, an heirloom engagement ring all have highly charged emotional significance for most of us. When I was an adolescent, an I.D. bracelet on a girl's wrist meant that she was a social success because she and a guy were "going steady." A girl and a boy would exchange class rings to indicate that they were a couple.

Jewelry worn in earlier times can tell us much about the people who wore it. Centuries ago, mandarins enclosed their very long nails in silver and gold sheaths, not just for protection but to further emphasize their leisure-class status. I have a ring that my great-great-grandmother wore as a wedding ring on her marriage finger. As thin as my fingers are, it will only fit my

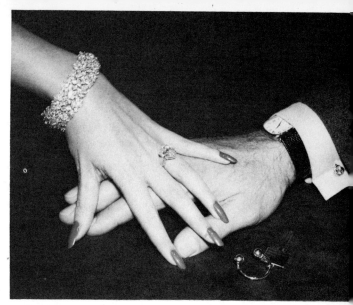

JEWELRY FROM TIFFANY

pinky. That means that seventy years ago a female ancestor of mine wore a size #2 wedding ring!

Status jewelry can be as obviously expensive as Elizabeth Taylor's diamonds, or as exclusive as a Harvard class ring. Rings bearing a family crest can serve as a tradition as well as a sign of social elitism. Wearing a ring on the little finger, or pinky, was once thought to be a sign of sexual hangups for females as well as males. And wearing more than one ring on one hand, which is now quite in vogue was thought to be rather garish, at best, years ago.

A ring worn on the third finger of the left hand means one is "taken." It is a symbol of either engagement or marriage. Most women and many men wear wedding rings. Women's wedding rings can be plain or encrusted with jewels, while men almost always wear plain gold bands. Before the sexual revolution, unmarried women who traveled with men often wore a ring from the five-and-ten to avoid the fish eye of the hotel clerk.

Engagement rings traditionally are worn by women to indicate that they are going to be married. The ring may be an heirloom with an old-fashioned stone in an antique setting, passed down from generation to generation, or a very modern solitaire diamond. Although engagement rings are usually worn only by the bride-to-be, the ring's observable value often becomes a highly visible assessment of her intended's financial status, or at least how much he values their betrothal.

JEWELRY SELECTION

Most of us wear some jewelry, even if it is just a watch or a wedding ring. The rules of jewelry selection are simple enough, but we are often led astray by fads.

Rule #1: As in clothes, the more you can subtract and still get the effect you want, the more successful your look will be. Although it is currently fashionable to wear lots of trinkets, the best look is achieved by eliminating as much excess baggage as possible. Charlotte Ford is never laden down with lots of rings and bracelets. It's one or two important pieces—and that's it. Avoid the Liberace overkill.

Rule #2: If you are large-boned (but not necessarily tall) and large-featured, you can wear more massive pieces than if you are small-boned.

Rule #3: If you are lucky enough to have nice jewelry for your hands, please keep it clean. Nothing looks richer than shiny stones and gleaming gold, or even silver.

RING REACTIONS

If a handsome ring turns your finger green, do not assume you have had a fake palmed off on you. Fourteen- and even eighteen-karat gold metals contain alloys that can cause this chemical reaction on certain skins. Try coating the inside of the ring or bracelet with clear nail polish.

Some rings, especially wide bands, can appear to be causing a reddening condition around the finger. Actually, the skin has been sensitized by irritants—your dishwashing detergent is a common culprit—which have been prevented from drying properly under the ring. The rubbing of the ring against the skin can further provoke irritation. Take the ring off and, if it is gold, platinum or silver, sterilize it. (Don't sterilize pearls or such semiprecious stones as opals.)

To sterilize, gently simmer in one cup water to which a tablespoon of detergent has been added. Turn off flame after five minutes and let cool.

GLOVES

In my earliest memories of Easter morning, my mother always draped a fresh new pair of white cotton gloves over the basket of goodies left outside my door as an extra gift from the Easter Bunny. I realize now that she was making sure that I had a fresh clean pair that fit. While gloves were once worn by the upper classes in all seasons, today they are rarely considered a social requirement except at a debutante ball. Long evening gloves are the trademark of cabaret chanteuse Hildegarde, who even plays the piano with them on. She removed them once to perform a serious musical piece composed by her beloved piano teacher, Isador Ackron, who had recently died. In tribute to him, she played his piece "nude" from the elbows down. The reviewers praised her musicianship, but the headlines read "Hildegarde has hands!"

Gloves can be beautiful, elegant, protective and convenient, but they don't always take you everywhere, as I learned several years ago. For some time I had been plagued by sun poisoning on, of all places, my hands. When I finally decided not to be at the mercy of the sun, I took to sunbathing in white cotton gloves worn with a very tiny bikini and white sun hat. This eventually set a trend at conservative old Quogue on New York's Long Island although initially the subject of much conjecture and ridicule by those who wore white gloves just about everywhere but at the beach. Gradually, however, it became actually fashionable to sport gloves while sunning. Many of the ladies summering and suffering had had their liver spots chemically removed and were happy to have an acceptable way to protect their skin from further exposure.

HAND IN GLOVE:
A FEW HISTORICAL FACTS

Although it is believed that cave dwellers used a primitive form of glove for protection, it wasn't until the thirteenth century that ladies started wearing gloves as adornments. These were elbow length and were made of linen. Pontifical gloves and those worn by royalty have always been elaborate and costly, often encrusted with jewels. Some gloves leave the fingers free (as those worn by knights in shining armor, and some bridal gloves).

All of us should wear gloves for winter sports such as skiing and ice skating—one can even buy gloves with battery-operated warmers! I like wearing several layers of gloves. Mittens are even better, because the body heat from your hands and fingers accumulates more easily. In extremely severe temperatures, as I experienced one winter while vacationing at a Canadian ski resort, try thin plastic work gloves under your other layers. They help to keep the body heat in.

I wear gloves for summer sports to protect them from aging and drying effects of the sun, as well as to prevent calluses. I cut the fingertips off my tennis gloves so that my nails won't be subjected to the pressure of play, or to perspiration acids. However, many women will want to keep their nails relatively short for the summer months. Nails grow a lot faster during the warm weather and look especially healthy then, regardless of length.

●

"I have tongue depressors in the fingers of my glove so they won't bend, to avoid breaking a blood vessel or straining a finger. But I take the padding out of the heel of my glove so I can 'feel' the ball better."

—BUCKY DENT, Yankee,
Baseball's 1978 MVP

●

"The sabre fencer's glove extends halfway up a fencer's arm. You look for leather that fits well around the sleeve because, although there is padding around the top part, you want the glove to fit as closely as possible to reduce the possibility of an opponent making a 'touch.' "

—STEVE KAPLAN, Olympic fencer

•

GLOVES AS PROTECTION

Men as well as women find it necessary to protect their hands against dirt, dust, the strong alkalis in detergents, typewriter ribbon, carbon, paint stripper, and even against the clinging odor from chopping onion and garlic. For an extra beauty treat while you are working, apply hand lotion and/or cuticle cream before you put on your gloves. Your body heat increases the softening action of the creams. The very best way to help these creams along is to wear washable cotton gloves under rubber gloves. Film editors' gloves are thin, cheap enough to be dispensable, and therefore perfect for this purpose.

Caution: Remove the gloves at least every hour and rinse your hands in cool water. Otherwise your nails may soften and be more susceptible to breakage.

The Many Ways
to Make You Handsome

JUST LOVE IT when people say, "Linda, you must do nothing but stay at home and take care of your hands." I am not only raising two boys, but I also pitch in and do the housework. Many of my competitors live in cotton, so to speak, but I refuse to. I had a decision to make: to be supercareful of my hands or be a mommy. I decided you don't get many cracks at motherhood, so my solution was easy. That was nineteen years ago, and I haven't lost a job yet, even to younger competitors.

Greg Fortune, the leading male hand model, told me, "I built a whole goddamned house to prove I could do it and still be the world's most photographed male hands!" In fact, the more you work with your hands, the faster your nails will grow.

Piano playing and typing actually increase the rate of growth. *Note:* Women who want to keep their long nails and still type and play the piano can try applying a little strip of masking tape over the nail tips for protection.

In addition to stimulating nail growth and manual dexterity, there is nothing like manual activity to work off aggression and nervous tension. I have completed many a needlepoint canvas on the energy of pent-up frustration and anger. There is a wonderful release in deliberately sticking a needle into something (a canvas rather than a person). Former football star Rosy Grier has been known to sew a fine needlepoint from time to time. You want to use a thimble to protect your nails and fingertips. Working with clay is another wonderfully expressive way of not only increasing dexterity but also releasing inner rage.

I love to garden. Although my gardening activities are confined to houseplants, I find few activities as rewarding as planting seeds and watching them grow. I use gloves so I can dig in. If you don't like to wear gloves, draw your nails across a bar of soap to protect them from dirt and splinters that could become imbedded in the nail base.

Cooking can be wonderfully creative for men as well as women. Cutting and slicing are great tension reducers. Kneading dough is even better. You can wear gloves for these chores to protect your hands from odors, stains, cuts, etc. I love raw garlic. It completely agrees with my insides, but by contrast, crushed raw garlic can make the backs of my fingers red and sensitive. So I wear gloves when handling it.

If you don't use gloves, take care to rinse your hands a lot while cooking. Some vegetables can stain the hands and nails. Keep lemon and water handy in a squeeze bottle (one tablespoon lemon juice to one cup water) to rinse hands with. Or substitute vinegar for the lemon. A wedge of lemon covered with cheesecloth will remove odors as well as stains when rubbed on the hand.

Take extra care when at the stove and always use pot holders to prevent burns.

If you do burn yourself, apply an ice cube immediately to the burn. Keep a good burn ointment in a convenient place. Vitamin E capsules often aid in speedy healing. If you have a really bad burn, see your doctor, of course.

SPORTS

Sports activities keep the hands, as well as the whole body, in condition. Just remember that the backs of the hands are especially vulnerable to aging and drying because of sun exposure. Unlike your face, they are not usually thought of as needing extra protection. Actually they are more often exposed than other parts of the body. Most of us will remember to wear a hat to keep the sun off our heads before we reach for gloves to protect our hands. To prevent dryness, aging and freckles:

1. Apply a protective sun screen often.
2. Apply moisture lotion after washing.

•

SPORTS STARS DIFFER IN ATTITUDES
TOWARD PROTECTING THEIR HANDS

Jim Dietz, U.S. Olympic champion single sculler, told me, "I'm very careful not to jam my fingers during a season. I don't play basketball. Actually, I don't even mess around with a Frisbee!"

While most pro football players have to endure painful stinging hands during hours of exposure to the cold during a game, I would never have imagined cold weather to be a factor to be reckoned with in golf. However, PGA star Tom Watson told me, "We don't move around like tennis players, and cold weather can be a problem. And when you play a tournament like I did in Kansas, the guy who makes the big money is the one who can keep his hands warm." Watson, who holds the world record for banking the most money in the history of the tour, must be keeping his hands very warm.

Although Rod Gilbert, high goal-scorer for the Rangers hockey team, credits as much of his success to his manual dexterity as to physical strength (enabling him to perform superior stick handling and shooting), he thought my inquiry about how he protected his hands rather amusing. He told me, "Although we, of course, wear gloves, hockey is such a rough sport that nothing else seems very hazardous."

SPECIAL PROBLEMS

Pregnancy

During pregnancy the skin is drier and may be more sun-sensitive, so pour on the hand lotion and sun-block creams. On the other hand, nail growth flourishes, so use your longer nails to draw attention away from your changing body shape. Your fingers may swell, so make sure your rings are large enough. Your hands will return to their original size (providing you don't retain a lot of extra weight), so while you're pregnant you might experiment with eye-catching, brightly colored, inexpensive costume jewelry.

Odors and Stains

Gloves are, of course, the preferred ounce of prevention. However, you can remove most odors and stains by rubbing the skin with a half a lemon—wrapped in cheesecloth if you want to be really efficient. Attack persistent stains like "smoker's finger" with a pumice stone dipped in lemon juice. (The best solution is a cigarette holder.)

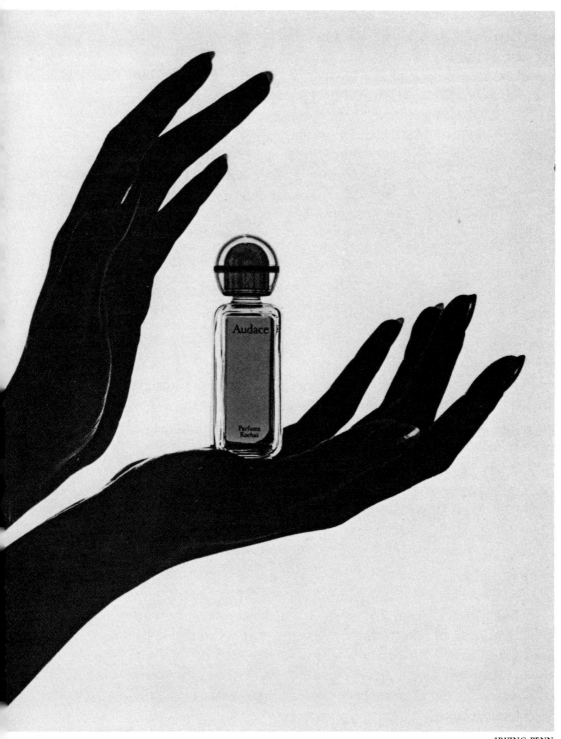

Audace

Parfums
Rochas

IRVING PENN

Remove stains under nails with an orange stick covered with cotton and dipped in hydrogen peroxide. If you don't get it all neatly clean, dip the cleaning stick in some Clorox. Don't let any dirt, as opposed to stain, remain under your nails, or you may develop a fungus infection.

Hair Removal

Women with excess hair on fingers and arms tell me they prefer waxing as the best method of removal. Most salons provide this service for a nominal fee, and the effects last from four to six weeks. I don't recommend that you try this at home, as the wax used has to be fairly hot to "grab" the hair, and few of us are ambidextrous enough to handle hot wax with the "other" hand.

Depilatories like Nair work well, but are pretty strong for the sensitive backs of hands. If your problem is mainly hirsute arms, Nair or a similar product can be a good bet. Just be sure to test yourself carefully for any possible allergies. Electrolysis, also available, is permanent but painful and very expensive.

•

TV CAMERA FIGHTS FUZZ (AND LOSES!)

Years ago, a copywriter on a commercial for watchbands was determined that anyone who sported one on TV would have hair-free wrists. I was chosen as the model, especially for my virtually hairless wrists. (How would you ever dream that anyone would love you for that particular quality?) During the actual filming, however, the director back-lit my hands— illumination which is always flattering to hands as well as faces, but which shows up every little detail because of its silhouette effect. After looking into the camera, the writer was no longer satisfied with the status of my wrists and begged me to shave them (I won't, but some hand models do), or use a depilatory (not on *my* untested little mitts). We compromised by cutting the hairs very close to the skin with a manicuring scissors.

Everyone was happy. When I saw the spot on the air, however, I was appalled. The closeup of the watchband so enlarged the area that the teensy hairs that remained on my wrist looked like a grass lawn that had just been attended to by a meticulous gardener!

●

HOLIDAYS

You want your hands to look as though you do nothing but lie on a couch and eat chocolates all day, and yet you may be performing marathon cooking, cleaning and gift-making tasks. During such hectic times, we all tend to let everything else go. Your hands deserve all the loving care they can get, and this is the ideal time to treat yourself to a professional manicure. Besides, someone may give you a gorgeous ring or a smashing watch on Christmas morning, and you will want to show it off to its very best advantage.

NAIL BITING

Over 50 percent of the people bite their nails at some point in their lives. Break the habit, for it can lead to acute infection and it can also shorten the nail bed permanently, which will result in a shorter "pink" section of the nail. Use tons of cream on your cuticles and skin so that the redness around your nails is lessened immediately. Wear gloves over the cream for at least one week to get you started. Keep cuticle and nail scissors handy to avoid biting or ripping off nails and cuticles. Clip ragged skin immediately and apply a dot of hydrogen peroxide with a Q-Tip. If possible, both men and women should use coat after coat of nail mender and wrappings. (see p. 107). Manicurist Nena Ricco reminds people to pay special attention during stressful times, like driving a car or watching an exciting movie, when biting is most likely to occur.

Is there a local self-hypnosis clinic nearby that gives habit-control therapy? Or perhaps it may help to write a paragraph describing how it feels to want to bite your nails, and also describe yourself resisting the temptation. Think of yourself with healthy hands and nails that you can show off to everyone. Visualize, at least three times a day, the more controlled you, the you who's on top of the habit. Reward yourself as you pass each of the seven days of the first week without biting or picking at your nails. Then reward yourself once a week. Treat yourself to a professional manicure as soon as the first week without nail biting is over.

Because your chances of breaking the habit get better as your nails begin to look better, this is the one time I recommend acrylic extensions. Nail biters have often damaged their nail bed already, so unless you have an allergic reaction to the acrylics, they are far preferable to the existing nail. Manicurist Hae Young in New York works wonders with men as well as women in getting former nail biters into good shape by applying acrylics.

The following is adapted from *Habit Control in a Day* by Nathan H. Azrin and R. Gregory Nunn (see Suggested Reading, p. 187):

10 STEPS TO STOP BITING YOUR NAILS

1. Try to keep hands away from the face and *notice* when you are biting. Watch yourself do this in a mirror and see what it looks like. You usually avoid facing what you do. See it clearly now.

2. List all the ways and situations in which you bite and when—e.g., on the telephone, watching TV, etc. Make a frequency chart that you keep faithfully for several days. You are going to observe yourself as if it were another person—clinically albeit lovingly.

3. When you bite, do it slowly and deliberately. This is so

that you will be able to consciously interrupt it, when you are ready to change it.

4. List all the inconveniences you experience because of your nail biting—e.g., hiding your hands, a reluctance to gesture freely, wearing less jewelry than you'd like.

5. Identify what you do immediately before biting.

6. Clench or grasp an object, like the arm of a chair, or a rubber ball, at these times.

7. Perform this grasping instead of biting procedure several times a day.

8. Return to the "inconvenience" list and indulge yourself with some terrific reward. Wear jewelry you wouldn't have thought acceptable on you before. Gesture grandly. Even compliment others on their hands (which is very brave because it will consciously call attention to your hands). Buy an electric manicure set.

9. Tell friends of your intention to stop biting your nails, so they can support you and reinforce your progress. Use someone you really care about, like a lover, or a manicurist who has been encouraging. Show them how you are coming along, and accept the praise.

10. *Give yourself a great big hand for breaking the habit!*

Special Treats
for Your Hands and Nails

*T*RY AT LEAST one of these treats every week for the best hands and skin you've ever had. If you are clearing up a severe problem like detergent hands, inflamed cuticles, or badly bitten nails and skin, use one of these treats daily, for immediate results.

1. Warm a small amount of olive oil in the top of a double boiler until tepid. (Make sure top of double boiler is dry before adding.) Apply to hands, nails, and especially to the skin around the nails. Put on cotton or plastic gloves for about ten minutes. Remove the gloves and massage the oil into your cuticle for another ten.

2. Treat #1, with wheat germ oil rather than olive oil, enriches the hands and cuticles with healthful vitamins.

3. Vitamin E seems to have a healing effect on inflamed skin. Follow the above procedure. I find the large vitamin E capsules perfect for this, as they are cheaper than bottled vitamin E. Also, keep some E capsules in the kitchen to soothe and heal kitchen burns and cuts.

4. Special delicious scrub and mask:

> 2 ounces liquid lanolin
> cold cream or any oil handy
> 1 tablespoon honey
> 1 egg yolk
> Enough almond meal to make a paste (or substitute dry oatmeal)

Work this into your hands and nails. Keep massaging for ten minutes, if you can. Then wrap a warm towel around your hands and let them "cook" for another ten. Wash off. This is a wonderful treat, especially for chapped or badly stained hands (for heavy stains, add one teaspoon of lemon juice). If you want this mixture to keep about three weeks in your refrigerator, add one tablespoon of tincture of benzoin which is available at drugstores. *Note:* this adds a slightly medicinal odor.

5. The pulp of a papaya is terrific for your skin. Hula dancers use papaya to keep their hands smooth. Working the pulp with the fingers also helps to keep them supple.

6. Watermelon pulp, too, is a fabulous skin softener. When making a fruit salad, save some watermelon for pulp and work it with your fingers. Rub into your hands thoroughly and then rinse. Your hands will feel like baby's skin.

EXTRA TIPS OR HANDOUTS

1. Don't use your nails to split pages open. Paper cuts are painful.

2. Don't use your nails to open jars or to scrape the lobster meat from the claws. If it's worth getting at, it's worth getting the proper utensil.

3. Use cooking tongs to remove hot foods or baby bottle from a boiling kettle. Keep pot holders (mitts preferably) handy in the kitchen, as well as first aid burn ointments.

4. Open jewelry clasps or lockets with a metal nail file rather than your nails.

5. Always use a pen or pencil to dial and use your knuckles to press for elevators.

6. Don't keep your hands in chemicals, or even hot water, longer than necessary. If you love to soak for hours in a hot tub, try to keep your hands out of the water as much as possible.

7. Moisturize your hands at least as often as your face.

8. Try to overcome such habits as putting your fingers in your mouth or picking at your polish. You can pick off a layer of nail as well.

9. Cover red hands with a little makeup. It's far better and easier than trying to hide them.

10. Wash your hair with the pads of your fingers rather than your nails. It's better for your circulation as well as your manicure.

11. If a friend is bedridden, consider presenting her (or him) with a professional manicure. Most good salons will provide this service for a reasonable fee.

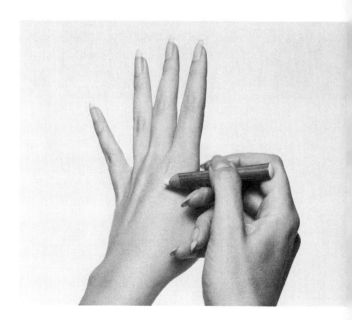

Spot stick to cover scars or freckles

HAND EXERCISES FOR STRONGER AND
MORE BEAUTIFUL HANDS

These exercises improve circulation and reduce tension.

1. Clench and release fists. This is especially effective if your hands are prone to that tingly pins-and-needles feeling. It works even better if you clench a rubber ball.

2. Let your arms and hands dangle limply at your sides and then shake them back and forth vigorously.

3. Rotate the wrists in circles, and shake your hands rapidly up and down. (Fig. 1)

4. Flick nails outward against the ball of your thumb. This will stimulate the nail matrix and improve circulation. (Fig. 2)

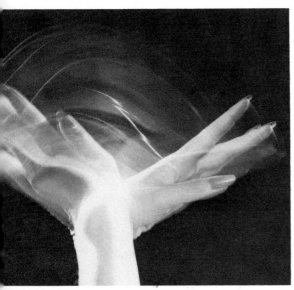 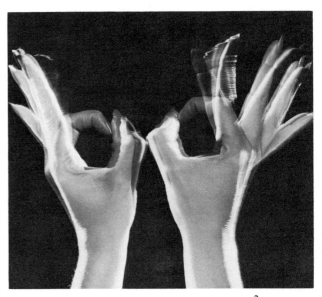

1   2

5. These next two exercises were taught to me by Tanao Sands, who studied dance, body harmonics and healing with Hawaiian masters (*kahunas*). In order to keep their hands supple, hula dancers would spread honey on the palms and insides of the fingers. They were required to work the hand clean, using the thumbs, and the exercise was not considered complete until

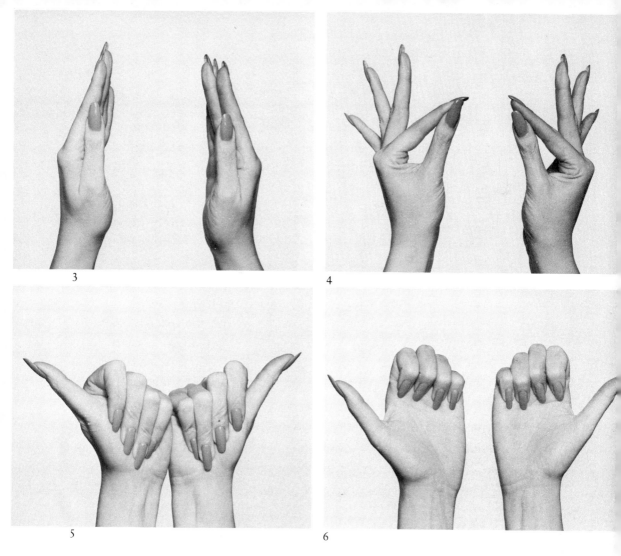

3 4

5 6

the hand was actually clean. So imagine you have spread rich, thick honey on your palms and the insides of your fingers. Work the honey off each of the fingers with your thumbs. When all the fingers are "clean," fold the fingers over the palms toward the wrists and "clean" the palm thoroughly with the fingertips, drawing the fingers up as far and as close as you can to the base of the fingers. (Figs. 3–6)

6. Bend your fingers back as far as they will go, straining till they almost tremble. Release. (Fig. 7)

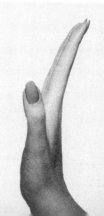

7

7. And now, for that old hand-model trick to (temporarily) reduce too-prominent veins on the back of the hand, shake hands vigorously and then hold them above your head for a few minutes. You are reversing gravity, and all the blood flows toward your arms and away from your hands, leaving them pale and smooth.

EMOTIONAL HAND EXERCISES

1. For increased will power: Practice keeping your thumbs out, i.e., away from your fingers. (Fig. 1) The thumb is the will and when you let it be covered with your other fingers, you are licked. Conversely, if you attend a meeting and see your opponent's thumbs in, you know you have him. So consciously keep your thumbs out.

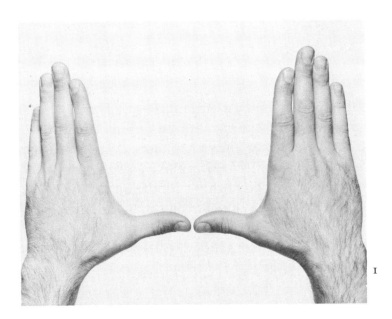

1

2. For flexibility of thought: Push the four fingers back, using the thumb of the opposite hand to brace them. (Fig. 2)

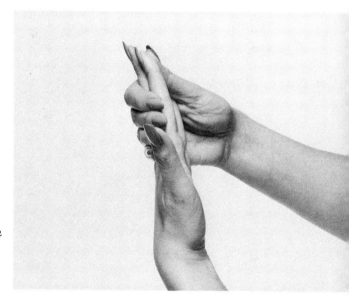

2

3. To release aggression and rage: Warren Robertson, eminent acting coach of such luminaries as Diane Keaton and Madeline Kahn, directs his students to thrust their hands in front of them forcefully, while shouting "No more!" or "Get Away!" to an imaginary person (but one toward whom you have worked up angry feelings). Really committing yourself to this, in the privacy of your own room, of course, can release an enormous amount of the pent-up aggression we all carry around with us.

4. If you are feeling sad, and tears won't come to give you release, Warren Robertson advocates that you stand with your arms outstretched in front of you with your palms down. Visualize someone you love or loved very much on the opposite wall. Move only your fingers as if you were waving "Bye-bye." The child in you responds with the release of tears.

Suggested Reading on Hands

Manwatching, by Desmond Morris. Harry N. Abrams, Inc., New York, 1977

Gestures, by Desmond Morris. Stein and Day, New York, 1979

The Book of the Hand, by Paul Tabori. Chilton Co., Book Division, Philadelphia, 1962

Habit Control in a Day, by Nathan M. Azrin, Ph.D., and R. Gregory Nunn, Ph.D., Pocket Books, New York, 1977

Body Language, by Julian Fast, Pocket Books, New York, 1970